Staying Alive

The Varieties of Immortality

Jason K. Swedene

University Press of America,® Inc.
Lanham · Boulder · New York · Toronto · Plymouth, UK

Copyright © 2009 by
University Press of America,® Inc.
4501 Forbes Boulevard
Suite 200
Lanham, Maryland 20706
UPA Acquisitions Department (301) 459-3366

Estover Road
Plymouth PL6 7PY
United Kingdom

Library of Congress Control Number: 2009932317
ISBN-13: 978-0-7618-4758-8 (paperback : alk. paper)
ISBN-10: 0-7618-4758-8 (paperback : alk. paper)
eISBN-13: 978-0-7618-4759-5
eISBN-10: 0-7618-4759-6

⊖™ The paper used in this publication meets the minimum
requirements of American National Standard for Information
Sciences—Permanence of Paper for Printed Library Materials,
ANSI Z39.48-1992

FOR MY PARENTS

Contents

FOREWORD

By Dr. Ryan Vaughan, Binghamton University

Jason Swedene is immortal. There, I said it. When we think about the concept of immortality, most of us conjure up images of the fountain of youth or Walt Disney's cryogenically frozen head, or better yet, Thor and his titan of a hammer. That's about where it ends, but that ending is a purely linguistic one. An end bound only by the limits of language in that we all generally agree that "immortality" means "to never die," and this is where Swedene's work begins.

I see this book being as much about language as it is about philosophy, for Swedene seeks to expand our accepted definition of immortality to encompass all the nuances and offshoots that spring forth from a multitude of linguistic interpretations. We have been conditioned by our culture, our environment, and our media to frame our lives as a series of binaries: black/white, male/female, Republican/Democrat, Yankees/Red Sox, assuming there isn't, or refusing to acknowledge that there is, something in between. It's this kind of thinking, one-dimensional and close-minded, that can often impede our progress, beginning with the individual and ascending to blanket the entire culture or society. The concept of immortality is no different. It gets shuffled into the binary deck as alive/dead, and if you're not one, you're certainly the other. This book looks to expand on our understanding of life and death by proliferating a whole host of possibilities in between these two spectrum ends, and possibly suggesting that these aren't, in fact, the ends at all. For me, this work presents immortality like a classic Ali/Frazier title bout. The public viewed Ali as the ultimate purveyor of the "sweet science": quick, agile, effortless. Frazier was the bull, using raw power and basic technique to bludgeon opponents. Together, they represented opposite ends of pugilistic engagement, but to assume or believe (as many people had been conditioned to) that Ali lacked power and Frazier lacked grace is as ridiculous as me stepping into the ring with either of them. By the same token, to believe that there is nothing shared between life and death, before and beyond, is remiss and irresponsible.

This is a rather complicated undertaking. One (me) might even view it an arduous task considering the religious/spiritual implications alone, that immortality suggests. Swedene does not shy away from what can often be a fruitless discussion. Religion, when thrust into public discourse, so often disintegrates into a "my God can kick your God's ass" shouting match, but Swedene plays the role of moderator here with the calming voice and aplomb of a skilled therapist or salesman, depending on how you look at it. Under the umbrella of immortality, he is able to present each unique and specific religious doctrine with respect to immortality without establishing a theological hierarchy, but rather, accepting a variety of beliefs as part of a search that is perhaps more consequential than the beliefs themselves. In other words, the desire to rethink our notion of "immortality" should transcend petty religious squabbles and regard those differences as beneficial to informing this dialogue.

Swedene writes with a ferocious veracity that leaves no man behind. I've read too many books where the genius author is speaking only to his (pardon my lack of gender equality) two or three genius buddies who meet once a week to drink snifters of brandy and make fun of state schools. What good is genius if it can't be efficiently relatable and understood by the populace; just ask Bill Gates about Windows Vista if you think I'm a lunatic. Swedene takes the complex and intricate concepts that inform his arguments and delivers them in a frank and seemingly extemporaneous manner that draws in even the most reluctant reader. His writing does not rest on the laurels of arcane philosophical references and citations. It is fully aware of its connection to mythology, psychology, religion, politics, pop culture, literature, theory, art. There's a passion to his writing that gives the book the warm feel of a good novel as opposed to the cold antiseptic feel of a text book. The job of simplifying the intellectual without pandering to the lowest common denominator is a challenging one. Too many have tried and failed, but Swedene is both humble and skilled enough to pull it off. If a book is read in the woods, and no one can understand it, is it really a book?

What registered most with me is Swedene's realization that we have very little to do with establishing our own individual immortality. We can try all we want, but like many other cultural and philosophical phenomenon, most of its legitimacy and longevity are determined by others. This elicits interesting questions about the pursuit of immortality in its various forms. Our distance from determining it should reduce our obsession with it, but such is not the case. Many of us, whether consciously or not, are consumed by "living on" despite how arbitrarily immortality is determined. I liken it to an artist too consumed with how his or her work will be received. Once the artist anticipates a reaction, and subsequently changes his or her vision to accommodate that reaction, the slope becomes slippery. Soon, the vision is overwhelmed and eventually compromised by seeking to assuage any and all elucidation. It's an exercise in extreme futility that can be debilitating. Similarly, the pursuit of preserving immortality is akin to living your life for others. The more you try to manipulate your life according to what you think others might remember and preserve, the less pure and "real" your experiences are. The irony of that last statement being in a book about immortality that will arguably make its author immortal is not lost on me, but that's part of the book's charm. Swedene doesn't make the book feel like his own personal attempt to be immortalized. That's what his introspective brand of song writing is for.

I went to college with Jason Swedene, and we were in a band that he fronted. The Jungle Monsters, in case you were wondering. I spent countless hours singing his words along with him in dorm rooms and sparsely attended local venues. His songs are heartfelt, critical, and relevant... not unlike his academic writing pursuits. What I learned about him through his songs and living with him has stayed with me over the past sixteen years, so I suppose he has already gained a modicum of immortality, even though he would surely argue that the amount of immortality one achieves is moot, you either have it or you don't. We used to play an innocent game called "Swedene vs. The World." Every time something unfortunate would happen to Jason: tripping on his own feet, putting his foot in his mouth, dropping a freshly made bowl of pasta on the floor, we would tally one for The World. World – 1, Swedene – 0. He could gain points by having a particularly good idea or getting through the day without inadvertently offending someone. The competition was fierce, and I don't even remember what the score was; probably because the game is still going on, and this book has certainly leveled the playing field, if not tipped the scales in his favor. The reason I mention this triviality, is to at once humanize the brilliant author of this book and point out that we're all playing the same game of "Us Vs. The World," and no matter what the final score is, our immortality remains unchanged.

Ryan Vaughan
Binghamton, N.Y.

PREFACE

This book, to modify Galileo's words, is not about how one achieves immortality but about what kinds of immortality one hopes to achieve. Although there seem to be those who authentically seek to be fully extinguished upon death, there are less who authentically desire to have nothing they worked on survive, and still less who would most prefer to be completely forgotten. This book is for all those who have thought about continued existence in any of its forms including progeny, memory, legacy, paradise, prolongevity, and merging with more powerful entities.

. . .

I remember offering a course in the Philosophy of Immortality, called 'The Varieties of Immortality,' in 2006, and I was shocked that student registrations for the course were maxed out within a week of open registration. What is it about my course in immortality that resonated with these inquiring young minds?

Could it be the teacher? I felt flattered at the thought.

The universality of the theme? Everyone has thought of it.

The interdisciplinary themes: history, aesthetics, science, philosophy, religion? Yes, the allure of immortality has shaped each of these.

My speculation was abruptly silenced when I heard that many of the students expected a class in the varieties of *immorality*!

. . .

Of the many books on the subject, many in print now tend to lean heavily on religious understandings of immortality. That is, on the immortality of the soul. There are also the books that are laden with philosophical jargon, which can at times make learning the language of the books a study in itself. As far as I know, there are no books which offer a subject-divided approach into the various forms of living forever. Most aspirants of immortality can form a hierarchy of the modes they would most prefer. As selfish as it sounds, I know I want them all. I leave it to the readers to determine what, if any, is the mode most worth seeking for them.

The way the book unfolds is to introduce thoughts on death, of course, as a gateway to thoughts on immortality. Closely behind thoughts of death are thoughts of love, which seeks its own continuation. From there, we have the continuation of memory: fame, and the continuation of the objects we leave behind: creative legacy. After creative legacy, I explore the concepts of spiritual immortality and prolongevity. Next, I examine how the idea of merging with non-Self is indispensable for immortality.

This book is not organized as a hierarchy or a reverse hierarchy of the varieties of immortality. It is arranged in a half-conscious, half-freely associated unveiling of the new concepts suggested by the previously explored ones. For example, readers will readily see that many forms of fame (renown) are possible because the famous have left objects or ideas behind to be scrutinized and enjoyed long after the famous have died. Fame and creative legacy seem good partners of sequence. All chapters are linked in this way and I allow the thoughts of each chapter to lead, as seamlessly as possible, into the next.

My aim has been, simply, to write a readable book that will afford the reader an increased sensitivity to the many ways the desire for immortality has shaped history, philosophy, art, and literature. Moreover, it is my sincere hope that each reader will adopt a sustained self-examination to inquire about this desire's manifestations in his own life. There is a companion website to this book, which contains links and pictures of note and interest. It is *http://www.lssu.edu/faculty/jswedene/immortality*.

Jason K. Swedene
Sault Ste. Marie, MI
March, 2009

ACKNOWLEDGEMENTS

This book underwent not less than two major waves of revision. Klaus Hergt, M.D., Thomas Noonan, Margaret Swedene, and Dr. James Zukowski were incisive readers who helped me arrange the chapters, offer tighter arguments, and adopt a new (and I believe, improved) tone. To all those, including Dr. Daniel T. Dorrity, who have graciously indulged my interest in the prevalence of immortality-chasing in the humanities, my acknowledgements. Thanks also to Lisa M.H. Sanderson and Tessa A. Clardy who identified and solved many of my formatting issues in the final days before the book went to press. Of course, any content errors and formatting mistakes are due to my oversight and do not reflect on the generosity and competence of the reviewers.

My gratitude is extended to the honors students of Lake Superior State University. These students, whose backgrounds and interests are quite diverse, reviewed this book throughout its stages and offered informed perspectives. They could be counted on to keep me focused on the book's real audience: thinking human beings, rather than merely those thinking beings with a background in the humanities. I received many helpful commentaries and editorials from these students, and I am continually appreciative of the curious group of students surrounding me.

Thanks lastly to my supportive parents who have given me life and, therefore, the opportunity to pursue immortality in all its forms. If the pursuit is ultimately elusive or illusory, the precious thrill of a mortal life would still far exceed the alternatives.

CHAPTER ONE: DEATH

Let us imagine a number of men in chains, and all condemned to death where some are killed each day in the sight of others, and those who remain see their own fate in that of their fellows, and wait their turn, looking at each other sorrowfully and without hope. It is an image of the condition of men.—Blaise Pascal, *Pensees*, #199.

The syllogism he had learnt from Kiesewitter's Logic: 'Caius is a man, men are mortal, therefore Caius is mortal,' had always seemed to him correct as applied to Caius, but certainly not as applied to himself. That Caius-man in the abstract-was mortal, was perfectly correct, but he was not Caius, not an abstract man, but a creature quite, quite separable from all others. He had been little Vanya, with a mamma and papa, afterwards with Katenka and with all the joys, griefs, and delights of childhood, boyhood, and youth. What did Caius know of the smell of that striped leather ball Vanya had been so fond of? Had Caius kissed his mother's hand like that? Could Caius preside at a session as he did? 'Caius really was mortal and it was right for him to die; but for me, little Vanya, Ivan Illych, with all my thoughts and emotions, it's altogether a different matter. It cannot be that I ought to die. That would be too terrible.' Such was his feeling.—Leo Tolstoy, *The Death of Ivan Illych*.

If you are reading this, no one has yèt to prove your mortality. Yet overwhelming empirical evidence of other human beings' lives and deaths leads you and I to face up to the fact that our ends are coming. Thus, Martin Heidegger (1889–1976 CE) was correct to point out that we are indeed beings-toward-death, and we ought to acknowledge it.[1] Death remains that event out in front of us as long as we exist, and contemplating it is a worthy exercise in being human. We carry our deaths with us as a birthright. Human beings are more or less conscious of their impending ends, although many have tried to distract themselves from it, because to die, I mean to *really* die, would indeed be "too terrible."

Throughout the millennia, much of human activity may be identified as a procession of attempts intended to mitigate death's consequences and, in some cases, to mitigate death itself. The early epic protagonist Gilgamesh (c. 2700 BCE) of the epic *Gilgamesh* (c. 1700 BCE) seeks to avoid it; Alexander the Great (c. 345 BCE) seems to have spent many hours contemplating his future fame; early Christians (c. 125 CE) saw death as something to be overcome (as Jesus overcame it); many Medieval peasants (c. 700 CE) believed heaven held the true happiness hitherto unattainable and death was necessary but conquerable; the towering figures of the Renaissance (c. 1450 CE) sought fame and legacy through enduring scholarship and creation, and a share in the eternal benefits of their Christian religion. The moderns (c. 1600 CE) attempted to align themselves with enduring, natural principles such as science and freedom. The early psychoanalysts (c. 1900 CE) attempted to expose our longing to live forever as narcissism. People of the ages have sought to mitigate death, and we, in our own age, are quite comfortable choosing from a menu of immortalities to create our own eclectic escape from inevitability. One chooses fame and legacy, while another chooses children and heaven. The early 21st century truly reflects this book's subject matter: the varieties of immortality. What we pursue, to be sure, is influenced by the past procession of attempts yet it is undoubtedly freely chosen for the needs of the present.

GILGAMESH AND THE BLACK DEATH

Cuneiform tablets pieced together tell a rich and evocative tale of one man's search for everlasting life. *Gilgamesh* is the earliest epic known to civilization (the story itself probably is more than four millennia old), and its insights into immortality have import far beyond its plot of a mortal undergoing struggles, facing danger, and defying enemies. When Gilgamesh rejects the amorous advances of the goddess Ishtar, Ishtar pleads to her father to kill Gilgamesh in retaliation for humiliating her.[2] Her father, in the fashion of all of the irrational gods of the day, agrees to send down the Bull from Heaven to make Gilgamesh pay for the offense against Ishtar. But unforeseen to Ishtar and her father, Gilgamesh and his friend Enkidu manage to kill the bull before it visits upon them Ishtar's retaliatory brand of capital justice. Now that the bull has been killed, Ishtar and the gallery of Mesopotamian gods and goddesses have been humiliated all the more. Anger and indignation lead them to afflict Enkidu with an illness that would gradually weaken Enkidu, make him bedridden, and ultimately kill him.

At this point in the story one wonders why Gilgamesh's friend's death is severe enough penalty for the divine humiliation. Why not just kill off Gilgamesh? Isn't one's own death the ultimate penalty?

To answer this, we have to consider what death is when it arrives. It is indisputably true that we human beings can meaningfully ponder death (even if some of us do not), but it is also true that it is impossible to understand the implications of non-existence. When we *might* finally experience non-existence, we do not exist anymore to ponder the horrors of death. Epicurus (341–270 BCE), the Hellenistic philosopher and champion of a restrained hedonism, once wrote that when the subject exists, death does not and when death exists, the subject does not. *I* never experience death, because when death arrives, the *I* is extinguished. When I lose my keys, I bear the loss. When I lose my life, I do not bear any lose because I do not exist. This point is at the forefront of artist Damien Hirst's (b. 1965 CE) mixed media image of a preserved, deceased shark in a casketesque box. When we "experience" death, it is of someone or something else and we are not dead. As long as we live, death is physically impossible.[3]

The claim for Epicurus, as for Damien Hirst, amounts to more than the claim that we cannot conceive of our own death because we are living. It is that death itself is never a reality for the living. This idea leads Epicurus to say that we should not try to conceptualize the inconceivable and worry about what is not reality. It also led Sigmund Freud (1856–1939 CE) to reason that this inability to conceive death is responsible for the shared delusion of immortality. According to Freud,

> It is indeed impossible to imagine our own death; and whenever we attempt to do so we can perceive that we are in fact still present as spectators. Hence the psycho-analytic school could venture on the assertion that at bottom no one believes in his own death, or, to put the same thing in another way, that in the unconscious every one of us is convinced of his own immortality.[4]

Thinking about our own death, a death which will occur at a future point, can cause immense anxiety *now*, but our death would result our becoming a non-being, and non-beings are of course incapable of pondering finitude and its supposed discontents. How could a non-being be capable of anything whatsoever? There are no discontents to be pondered by the dead. Finitude is only a problem for the living.

Why, then, does our impending death bother us so much? I think that one must consider an answer not quite suggested by Epicurus or Hirst, but nevertheless made understandable by their concepts. Epicurus: I do not exist when death exists. Hirst: death is a physical impossibility when one is living. We may even add Rene Descartes' (1596–1650 CE) observation: as long as I think, I exist. In my view, when we think about death, we are in the world of concepts, since the reality does not yet exist. In our minds, the "I" exists as the subject term and "death" exists as the predicate term. What makes Epicurus's dictum so difficult to acknowledge and glean solace from is that, *in thought*, the self and death do indeed exist at the same time *as a thought*. This thought creates the anxiety, and many of us *can't bear to think it*.

So, returning to Gilgamesh's punishment, what would be most proper consequence to "fit" the "crime" of Gilgamesh's insolence towards the gods—his own death, or the death of another? With his own death, he would not suffer emptiness, disappointment, or anything at all. He would be in Epicurus's world of reality, a world in which the self and death do not coexist. If another died, someone Gilgamesh loved, Gilgamesh would be around to endure the weight of his loss. He exists and so does death: the death of his beloved friend. He would be in the conceptual world where the "I" and "death" coexist. He cannot accept the thought of it. This is a severe punishment and, in terms of *his* feeling of the loss, it is more painful than Gilgamesh's own death.

Enkidu's death leads to Gilgamesh's anxiety about his own demise. It brings knowledge of death out of the abstract into the experienced (although, to experience the death of another is quite different than experiencing one's own death).[5] For Gilgamesh, the death of Enkidu brings his own mortality to the forefront. Gilgamesh's death is only postponed. It will happen later, but it will happen. A human being's life can be spared at one moment, but only until some later point in time. Gilgamesh, in fact, is so distressed about his own impending death that he begins a futile search for immortality. But he does not search for a spiritual life-after-death in the way that a pious believer would. Rather, he wants to never-die. He wants eternal youth and immortality on earth. He almost succeeds after obtaining a plant with the appropriate powers of prolongevity, but loses it to a serpent.

Gilgamesh marks the moment in literature in which humans' self-consciousness about death becomes movingly expressed. Self-consciousness about death must have emerged much before, but in the arts, this moment of its documentation is a watershed moment. We notice in it the features of what might be called the "cruel math" that concludes in the undeniable end of the one doing the equation. We awaken at some point to the problem of death. The problem of our deaths is not the "problem" of how to pay this or that bill or to fight on behalf of this or that cause. It is not to be dealt with within life. The problem involves life and yet is truly larger than life, if anything ever was. We seem so ill-equipped to deal with, let alone to solve, this problem. With our awakening to it, our attempted solution almost always takes the form of extending life or cheating death, whichever conception the would-be problem-solver prefers.

Consider when the Black Death, a combination of the bubonic, septicemic and pneumonic plagues, reached Europe in the fourteenth century. The lessons of *Gilgamesh* took on collective urgency, even though the urgency for each individual was, and is, ever-present.[6] An estimated twenty million people died. Many cities lost thirty to fifty percent of their populations. Statistics, though, do not get to the heart of the matter. On a mass scale, the living watched their beloved, their Enkidus, perish by the dozens. An Italian who lived through it, Giovanni Boccaccio (1313–1375 CE), wrote that it had caused even the seemingly unthinkable desertion of family members:

This scourge had implanted so great a terror in the hearts of men and women that brothers abandoned brothers, uncles their nephews, sisters their brothers, and in many cases wives deserted their husbands. But even worse, and almost incredible, was the fact that fathers and mothers refused to nurse and assist their own children, as though they did not belong to them.[7]

Formulated in *Gilgamesh* as one individual's sobering realization, and expressed in the Black Death[8] as a collective awakening, human beings' penetrating awareness of death is extraordinary, and this self-consciousness of the problem of death is the earliest step in seeking immortality in any of the varieties I shall discuss. The search for limitlessness begins with the realization of limit. My project concerns the postulates of immortality offered throughout the ages as responses to our intimations of this mortal "condition of men" that Blaise Pascal (1623–1662 CE) forcefully describes.

The condition is vividly depicted by the artist Francisco Goya (1746–1828 CE) in his *Executions of the Third of May, 1808*. Goya depicts a row of anonymous French executioners pointing their rifles at a man in a cruciform pose. Neither the Church in the background nor the lantern (symbolizing the 18th century Enlightenment) can stop the white-shirted man's death, which is to occur within moments. Those already killed are to the left of the picture. Those awaiting execution form a line behind the man. This is the condition of man even if many of us are lucky enough to go to our deaths without the violent drama of Goya's massacred.

Whether we have "gone" before, or will "go" sooner than later, or will tarry a while; all go. We know the end is coming, so then what? This book is about the *then what*. In particular, it's about the ways in which we have tried to maintain perpetual existence and influence. Ostensibly, responses vary and are often intertwined. The lover, the fame aspirant, the creator, the religious person, the prolongevity scientist, and the one who allies himself with the immortal to gain its strength can be one and the same person.

I shall now clarify the terrain of acceptable immortality (hell, then, is outside of this terrain), since thoughts about it may differ depending on the language one uses to express it and the perpetual experience one aspires to enjoy.

CONCEPTS OF IMMORTALITY

The careful thinker distinguishes clearly between words, concepts, and reality. Words are often used to express concepts, and reality sometimes elicits concepts; but words, concepts, and reality are distinguishable. For example, if I see the word 'HEAVEN,' I am led to ponder the meaning of what was said. If I died and my personality survives the experience and I see a Paradise, I affirm and alter my concept of heaven to suit its reality. In time, with honest thought, my concept would accord with reality. The letters 'H-E-A-V-E-N' are an arrangement of characters. The thought "HEAVEN" is not made up of characters; its content is meaning, which is understood. The place HEAVEN, if it exists, is a real thing separable from words used to describe it and thoughts intended to capture it.

A concept is a thought, which may have a connection to the real world. Whether concepts of immortality apply to the real world is arguable. People have differing beliefs about immortality (e.g., whether the subject's soul will live on in an afterlife[9]), and they also have conflicting beliefs on *what* one should do to attain the best mode of immortality. For instance, some seeking an afterlife have differed over whether God approves of just war or staunch pacifism. Pursuing actions of war and peace in accordance with God's will would presumably influence our chances of enjoying the best possible afterlife. (Again, the person in hell may be living forever, but this does not seem worth joyfully anticipating.)

But it is not the concepts themselves that cause disagreements, conflicts, and violence: concepts do not do that. It is those who adopt the concepts and seek to propagate them who struggle. People disagree and people commit violent acts based on internal motivations to attain the immortality that they believe in and value. It is the differing concepts, the belief in which inspires individuals to act in definitive ways, which I shall explore in this book.

One problem with any study of immortality considered as a *real* object of study is that those studying it have no first-hand experience of what they are studying. This is not a new problem to scholars, just ask natural theologians[10] and cosmologists[11], but it is a problem nevertheless. Because we have no first-hand experience of immortality, we students of immortality turn to revelation, experience, and evidence. Beliefs in revelation convince many to lay down their earthly lives to pursue eternal rewards. But, what of experience? I guess one could say we can *experience* evidence for an objective immortality and *experience* revelation for an objective immortality. Indeed, these experiences may be experienced so strongly that one might sooner doubt all information gathered through his senses than to doubt that someone speaks to him from on high. But such are first-hand experiences *of a description* of the afterlife and *of the described requirements* for attaining immortality. They are not first-hand experience of immortality itself. It comes down to, then, revelation and evidence. The revelation to Muhammad is the Muslim's evidence, and so on with believers of other faiths. Someone else's revelation becomes our evidence.

The experience of the evidence as interpreted by someone like humanist philosopher Corliss Lamont (1902–1995 CE) leads some thinkers to declare that real immortality an "illusion." But even these critics of the personal immortality thesis have no first-hand experience of non-immortality.[12] Nevertheless, the point of this discussion on experience, though, is not whether or not there is real immortality. Rather, it is whether we have first-hand experience either way, which we do not. Take the concept of fame-immortality. We experience others' fame. We may even experience our own renown. — Perhaps at this very moment the author of the latest *New York Times* bestseller is grinning, sipping mango-green tea, and glancing at a ceiling fan, contemplating her fame. But neither we nor that bestselling author experience our own fame-immortality, for the simple reason that we never fully grasp whether fame will be ours for all-time. Fame-immortality must be distinguished from social approval of our contemporaries. Whereas the latter may be experienced, the former may not.[13]

We have a cultural record of the varieties of immortality that humans believe are available to them. Those who articulate the concepts of immortality and those who chase after the dream of real immortality add to the human record of the varieties of immortality potentially available to each of us. That we relate to the varieties of immortality conceived by others gives others the ability to interpret, to add to, to refine, or perhaps, to reject them. In this book, readers will find an account of the concepts of immortality and their prevalence in Western Culture. Readers will not find accounts of what immortality, the real thing, is like. Yet I would go so far as to suggest that seeking immortality, however a culture or individual conceives of it, is perhaps the most significant impetus of human activity. This should not really surprise us. We know what life is like, most of us like life, we want it to continue, and if possible, we would prefer that our lives improve. These stances towards life and its quality lead to a desire for immortality.

SOME VARIETIES OF IMMORTALITY

Today, the most popular view of immortality in the West is the survival of the personality into the next life. The human being suffers physical death, but one's soul moves on to a place where it is far more vibrant and blissfully happy. Death occurs, of course, but death is not final: it is a door to a better life. "Death be not proud," John Donne wrote, for "one short sleep past, we wake eternally and death shall be no more."[14] El Greco's (1541–1614 CE) *Burial of Count Orgaz* painting even portrays the soul of a deceased count passing through a misty portal resembling a birth canal on its way to heaven. The lifeless body of the Count is being cared for by St. Augustine and St. Stephen at the bottom of the painting, yet just under the Virgin Mary, a midwife of sorts helps the vigorous spirit pass for its birth into the heavenly realm.

In the early western culture of Mycenae, there was a view of immortality as a spiritual one that was not necessarily a happy one. The Achilles of Homer's *Iliad* (c. 750 B.C.E.) proclaimed that he'd rather be a wretch on earth than king of the underworld. Homer's Mycenaean views of a shadowy, less-vibrant afterlife remained widely accepted through Classical Greece and beyond, even as its mainstream cultural influence was diminished, or at least transformed, by the increase of the Platonic and Christian traditions. Fame and legacy were the best of all possible outcomes for the Greeks.

Cultures influenced by Hinduism and Buddhism, cultures typically found in the East, believe that death may usher in an eternity of some other form of spiritual life, but it is not the continued life of the personality as it was on earth. In the case of Hinduism, the spiritual life hoped for is a loss of individuality and ego and a reunion with the divine. Short of attaining this release from the world (*moksha*), the Hindu banks on his spirit's continuation in another earthly being (*samsara*). With many Buddhists, the life hoped for remains a loss of individuality, but not a reunion with the divine. The new life is a state of blissful nothingness. Some Buddhists, in time, began to believe in a paradise more closely resembling the Christian and Muslim paradise. These views arose within the Mahayana sect.

Many hope that scientists, such as Aubrey de Grey, [15] will make possible earthly life without the necessity of dying. 'Prolongevity' is the fashionable academic term, but the attempt to cheat death is a strategy older than the nomenclature. The question of cheating death indefinitely, without limit, involves our ability to stop and reverse aging and disease. Along with speculations about the possibilities for such triumphs over our "condition" go the ethical considerations of whether we ought to be able to cheat death forever.

Those who do not believe in a spiritual immortality or hold out hope or intention that humans should not-die at all still subscribe to a material immortality, which is confirmed by theories on the indestructibility of matter. Yes, one's body ceases to be the unified whole that it once was, but it continues on forever in the sense that its raw materials are recycled indefinitely.

Or, if material immortality doesn't help one to find peace, there is always genetic immortality. The thinking is that our descendents get their lives and genetic codes from us, and so we live on through them and through successive generations carrying our genetic information. It is true that we spend much time discussing who babies and children resemble ("She looks like her mother," or "She looks like her grandmother when she was a baby"). Who cares that we see ourselves in the new generations? Is this just idle talk to fill the space of a boring family party? Or, perhaps is such talk indicative of the widespread acceptance that people live on through future generations?

We even talk of the "family name" continuing long after we depart this life. Monarchs, famously including Henry VIII, sought to have their family name and power survive through the birth of a certain kind of offspring (e.g., a son, or more specifically, a legitimate son). This immortality through legacy is mixed with procreative immortality.

Henry VIII also sought to magnify himself and his authority through paintings. In an age of increased printing distribution, a picture in which Henry looms asymmetrically large when compared to its background proves an aid to promoting prominence. Henry's self-aggrandizing evident in this portrait likely was in the same spirit as the one that spurred him to seek a legitimate son without showing moral reservations about committing betrayal, divorce, or murder.

Of course, family names need not be attached to genetic offspring. Former president Bill Clinton (b. 1946 CE), for instance, carries the name of an adoptive father, not his biological one. Nevertheless, a name signifies and evokes the legacy of the ancestors from that line.[16]

Then there is the concept of immortality we call fame. Fame, if it is orchestrated properly in ripe social conditions, can even sometimes outlast bloodlines. Artists create, generals conquer, and leaders change. Many have achieved fame in the process, and many more have strived for it. Some even orchestrate fame for others. A parent crusades for legal changes and social awareness following a child's suffering or death. Out of this we get things like Amber Alerts for missing children and Megan's Law, which mandates sex offender registration. A scholarship is created to honor a business student who embodied the ideals of service.

Add to this list the more personal, but no less humble, goal of leaving behind artifacts of our lives and creativity to future generations because we want our families to know who we were. Pictures, writings, a favorite hat, a wedding dress, a pocket watch: why bequeath them? Why care about their survival after we are gone? The goal of this immortality is not fame on a wide scope, but an intimate fame. As some secure the social recognition of anonymous others, some choose to secure that their family and friends recall them and "pay them mind."

WHAT DOES 'IMMORTALITY' MEAN?

The word 'immortality' certainly expressed different meanings to different people across different cultures, just as it expresses different meanings to many of us in our own time and place. We see some of these meanings (mentioned above) manifested more fully in certain cultures and times only to fade back in others. Often the cultural record maintains and emphasizes two or more concepts for an extended period of time. For instance, there is nothing mutually exclusive about Pope Julius II's (1443–1513 CE) desire for fame (the impetus for employing Michelangelo to work on his ambitious tomb) and the same pope's belief that his alert and self-aware soul would enjoy an afterlife in Heaven for eternity.

The Chinese emperor Qin Shi Huang (259–210 BCE) sought prolongevity into eternity (he kept trying elixirs designed to keep him alive forever), but realizing that the elixirs could fail (one of them, ironically, killed him), he had an army of terra cotta soldiers created to "guard" his tomb to keep his glorious burial chamber intact for perpetuity.

The different ways to pursue immortality share common qualities. I am most fond of the term 'indefinite' for characterizing the link between the various concepts of immortality. 'Indefinite' has at least two common meanings. The first is "imprecise" or "vague" as in the use "We have an indefinite amount of jelly beans left." The second meaning is "without clear limit" as in "You can stay at my home for an indefinite period of time." While it seems obvious that the second sense will be most relevant to immortality, the first sense is useful because the future we imagine and move into is always "imprecise" and "vague" since it is by definition ahead of us and numerically undefined.

Whether it is the Olympian gods who have numberless days, or the fame sought by Alexander the Great, or the 85-year-old cancer patient who undergoes another round of chemotherapy, all are guided in the hope that their lives and/or renown will remain ahead of the present. As Epicurus (341–270 BCE) put it, "The future is neither ours nor wholly not ours...we may neither count on it as sure to come nor abandon hope of it as certain not to be."[17] The future is indefinite from the standpoint of the present.

It is this indefiniteness that leads me to emphasize the love connection in immortality. Love, I argue, is a desire to extend a relationship on into the indefinite future. Love is always projecting itself into the future. The rational, decision-making, love vows its continuation into the future and the passionate, erotic love of the flesh seeks to secure a future in the passing on of life.

There is some uneasiness, philosophically, with how to understand the term 'immortality.' It seems that more than my notion of *living on indefinitely* is meant when we talk about immortality. For one thing, what does not have a *clear* limit may have a limit nevertheless. Think of summery weather. From a Northeast July perspective, the summery weather does not have a clear limit. It may come to an end by September 15, or it may continue on until October or later. We do acknowledge rightly, year after year, that there is a limit to summery weather. Whereas biological life and fame and physical creations left behind do not have clear limits concerning how long they will last, no one doubts that they have limits. Of course, one could argue that the Mausoleum at Halicarnassus *survives* still as stones, dust, memory, and legend. To this, it is quickly pointed out that the essence does not live on even if these other things do. It no longer stands as a unified whole.

What we may need, then, is an understanding of immortality that goes beyond the idea that the immortal person, place, thing, object, or idea *actually* exists without clear limit. We look for an immortal to exist without limit; however, this would be to seek in the real world an example of an immortal. But this is neither necessary nor warranted in a book about concepts of immortality, since, as I pointed out early on in this chapter, real world examples of the actually immortal cannot be found.

We do not need to find a real world example of an immortal to say something meaningful about the concepts of immortality, and the reason for this derives from the nature of knowledge and meaning. A conceptual piece of understanding need not correspond to the actual world to be epistemologically useful. The concept of a "chimera" has no examples (extension) in the real world, yet we can still talk about the concept's meaning (intension) and say things that are true about the concept even if the concept does not correspond to reality. "All chimeras are female monsters that have heads of lions and bodies of goats" is true because the concept "chimera" means "a female monster with a lion head and a goat body." The statement's truth does not depend on the concepts' correspondence to reality.[18] Chimeras don't exist, yet "all chimeras are female monsters that have heads of lions and bodies of goats" is true nevertheless. Similarly, the concept of "an immortal" need not have any real world examples to say meaningful things about the concept.

The prolific (but deceased) humanist Corliss Lamont wrote an informative book on the possibility of personal immortality in which he defines personal immortality as "the literal survival of the individual human personality or consciousness for an indefinite period after death, with its memory and awareness of self-identity essentially intact."[19] Lamont did not believe in an afterlife (and his book attempts to convince others of this position), but he nevertheless believes that "indefinite period after death" is an appropriate way to talk about the concept. Although for Lamont this concept has empty extension (i.e., it has no real world examples), the concept itself is meaningful and one may say meaningful things about it.

What makes the concepts of immortality worth studying is first the way that they motivate human activity and cultural trends and secondly, to help us, on an individual level, to choose or reject our own beliefs in immortality concepts after serious reflection of their merits. The "feel" of all immortality concepts is that there is no clear limit in sight, as the risk-taking teenager, the fame-seeking quarterback, and the promise-making lovers each could attest. I hope the pages ahead will succeed in bringing to the light the varieties of immortality, their major cultural antecedents, and the ways in which they continue to inspire human activity and trends.

We know that all humans die. We know that we are humans. We complete the syllogism in our minds; however, the syllogism is truly difficult to apply to our own individual person. We are like the Baroque painter Nicolas Poussin's (1594–1665 CE) Arcadians, who at a gravestone stand with bewildered faces that do not quite comprehend their predecessors' extinguished existences. They seem unable to fully understand their own mortalities. And we are like Ivan Illych who doesn't think the syllogism's combined premises "All men are mortal" and "Ivan is a man" apply to him, and who seems to perceive a cosmic injustice in the suggestion that it does apply to him ("That would be too terrible"). Being unable to complete the syllogism or unwilling to apply its conclusion, most of us want to continue on in some meaningful way.[20]

CHAPTER TWO: LOVE

And in the center of these is the goddess who guides everything; for throughout she rules over cruel birth and mating, sending the female to mate with the male, and conversely again the male with the female...First of all the gods she devised Love. —Parmenides

Eros [is] the most beautiful and immortal of the gods, who in every man and every god softens the sinews and overpowers the prudent purpose of the mind.—Hesiod, *Theogony*

In this chapter, I shall show how true love suggests an existence that continues into the indefinite future. This thesis is justified and made clear by many examples of poetry, philosophy, common sense, and common practice. Much of this chapter is focused on romantic love, although different forms of love such as love of God and love of friends would be covered by the claims made and defended. Love, for many Greek philosophers and their heirs, is divine and immortal. For example, Parmenides (approx. 520–450 BCE) considers it central a powerful force that influences universally (he claims that it "guides every thing"). Importantly, it is the inspiration for mating and reproduction. For his predecessor Hesiod (c. 775 BCE), love has a beginning, but no end. It exists indefinitely, without limit. Love in its divine personification (Eros) inspires humans to transcend their own biological finitude by having children and their own selfish myopias by finding joy in and through others. Love makes sense. For Hesiod, it is, overall, a rational plan without which the race would not continue. Yet, at the same time, Love is capable of thwarting and overtaking the plans we make for our individual lives: according to Hesiod, it "overpowers the prudent purposes of the mind."

As I shall point out often throughout this chapter, love strives for its continuation. Consider, for example, the ancient epic *Gilgamesh* (c. 1700 BCE), the oldest epic to come down to us in writing. His story is one of human yearning for a biological immortality[1], but Gilgamesh must settle for a lesser form. As the story unfolds, we notice that his frantic search for this earthly immortality *proceeds* from expectations of eternal love to considerations of earthly immortality and even creation-immortality such as architecture.

Gilgamesh rejects Ishtar's amorous advances, asking her rhetorically which of her lovers has ever received a permanent commitment from her. The answer is none. One ought not to bet on Ishtar's fidelity. Love, for Gilgamesh as it is for many of us, should never die. So, in the manner of a cross examiner who antagonizes his witness, Gilgamesh asks Ishtar:

What would I get if I marry you?
You are a brazier that goes out when it freezes,
A flimsy door that keeps out neither wind nor draught,
A palace that crushes a warrior,
A mouse that gnaws through its housing,
Tar that smears its bearer,
Weak stone that undermines a wall,
Battering ram that destroys the wall for an enemy,
Shoe that pinches its wearer.
Which of your lovers lasted forever?[2]

The poetry in the preceding quotation is telling: Ishtar habitually uses the intimacy of love as an inside track to wound, and ultimately, to dissolve the relationship. Shoes, for instance, are close to the feet and are supposed to provide benefits to feet as they walk the earth. Yet because of their closeness to the feet, they can also do harm to them. We might wonder why someone who loved Gilgamesh might try to undermine this relationship once it was forged. Perhaps Ishtar only seeks temporary amusement. Perhaps she seeks some other gain.

After musing in metaphors, Gilgamesh's final question to Ishtar presumes that love should last forever. And it assumes that Ishtar is not truly capable of loving forever. We may ask, then, why Gilgamesh should care that love lasts forever? Evolutionists would answer our question by saying that Gilgamesh, as male, wants to ensure that his genetic offspring will be nurtured by a faithful beloved and an unfaithful one would be less likely to nurture his offspring. He would also want to be close by the mother of his children to ascertain they are well-cared for: in short, then, he'd want the love to last for the sake of his genetic future.[3] Gilgamesh, of course, is a bit of a hypocrite. The author gives us the background of Gilgamesh's own sordid record: Gilgamesh "would leave no girl to her mother," neither "the warrior's daughter" nor "the young man's spouse."[4] Gilgamesh does not seem, even early in the text, like one who would have the time or motivation to devote himself to offspring! If the evolution model is correct, it is only part of the explanation for why Gilgamesh should demand lasting commitment. I set this answer aside for now.

Another answer for why Gilgamesh, or any one else, should care that love lasts forever is that the greatest tool to assess love's profundity and depth is the metric of longevity. On this view, longevity is not to be taken literally, but poetically: the terms 'forever' and 'eternal' are symptomatic of our inability to express the *depth* our feelings. So, we try our best making what is a "deep" feeling take on the words and meaning of feelings that are "long." It is not so much that we expect love eternal, but that our linguistic infirmities limit us to express depth in the terms of indefinite time. This view is perhaps best articulated by Johann Wolfgang von Goethe's (1749–1832 CE) Faust, who makes a deal with Mephisto to trade Mephisto allegiance in return for the full spectrum of human experience. Faust made this bargain because his lifetime of book learning could not instruct him in the ways of feeling. Reason was not enough. Love is an area that the reinvigorated Faust pursues. Mephisto accuses Faust of dishonesty when he learns that the now youthful and charming Faust intends to profess his love of Margaret. Mephisto sardonically sums up his thoughts on Faust's anticipated profession of lasting love:

> Oh wonderful!
> You'll swear undying faith and love eternal,
> Go on about desire unique and irresistible,
> About longing, boundless, infinite:
> That, too, with all your heart—I'll bet!"[5]

Faust responds that the words of love eternal are to express "an emotion of such depth, such turbulence" that when he tries "to find a name for it and nothing comes to mind," he expresses its "transcendent worth" as "eternal, yes, eternal, without end."[6] When our beloved loves us with a love that ends, we may conclude that they "didn't really love us after all," or at the very least, that they "didn't love us deeply enough."

True enough, many have lied using the words, "I love you" to express a lasting commitment only to secure a temporary gain. Yet even here, I believe that a manipulator can only benefit from the force of these words because the words do truly express some transcendent meaning: a transcendent meaning of continuation. The depth of the emotion and expectations of its resilience are inseparable. Depth and longevity become intertwined. The estranged lover could rightly ask: if the love is deep enough, why did you end the relationship?, or if you ended the relationship, did you ever really love me deeply enough?

LOVE AND THE FUTURE

So, what does love assume about the future? Lyricists and lovers everywhere profess "I'll love you forever," "I'll love you forever and a day," "I'll love you forever and ever."[7] Even "I'll love you until the end of time" suggests that the lover, who will probably expire before such the end of time itself, will nevertheless continue the love. Are such lovers being disingenuous? If not, why do such vows mean? It is possible that the professing lover may not have accepted his mortality. Perhaps the lover has accepted the inevitability of his death, but believes in a life hereafter in which the love will go on. But there is no theological reason why God would be committed to providing a forum for continued romantic love where there is no need for continued reproduction, and there seems good reason to conclude that the attentiveness a healthy relationship requires would distract us from enjoying the presence of God. In the Gospel of *Matthew*, Jesus says:

> You are mistaken, not understanding the Scriptures, or the power of God. 'For in the resurrection they neither marry, nor are given in marriage, but are like angels in heaven.'[8]

Jesus makes it clear that the focus of heaven is on communion with God and not the continuation of the lasting love expressed in the earthly institution of marriage. Jesus may be on to something here: there would be no need of procreation in heaven, and people would be at their happiest with their minds primarily on God.

Sometimes the actual practice of love does not last even when love is promised with genuinely committed hearts. People seem to mate like serial monogamists[9] rather than Catholics (to alter slightly Woody Allen's *Manhattan* quip that he thinks people should mate for life "like pigeons and Catholics"). Even though the practice of love in the contemporary world sometimes falls far short of the ideal, we would think it more than peculiar if one stated (sincerely) to one's beloved "I'll love you until I do not feel like it anymore." Some do have a litany of short-lived relationships and marriages: notoriously, many celebrities are included in this group, but the fact that they recommit themselves in marriage when so many in the past have failed speaks to the power of the concept of love eternal even when the lovers' love records speak to the concept of passing fancy.

Why remarry at all with unsuccessful, unsavory, or even horrible marriages in one's past? Marriage disregards the failed relationships of the past: it looks forward with hope and expectation that *this one* will last. We do seem intuitively more interested in our future experiences than in past ones.[10] Six failed marriages do not seem to threaten the seventh, so long as the seventh is the present one. Here we get a glimpse of the signals of immortality that lovers and lyricists express. Love is forward-looking and the future appears promising to well-intentioned lovers.

LOVE, FOREVER, AND CHANGE

Many say that nothing lasts. Even oak trees (that outlive family trees) eventually decay and die. The weather, hair color, clothing styles, governments, geography, and languages all change. So, what does it really mean *to last* when our lives are inundated with things that do not? It seems to me that when we say that this or that thing will last, what we mean is that it will be available to us as long as we need it. For example, a can opener that lasts is one that serves us well in opening cans every time we go back to the drawer to pull it out. But can openers that last are not like love that lasts. Perhaps sadly, the can opener has no say in its being used as such and has no recourse to get out of the arrangement.

In love, there are two different consciousnesses involved. Love is a relationship that is reciprocal with each person simultaneously acting as the lover and beloved. It is not like "loving" golf in which the sport is the beloved but never the lover. But the failure of one of the lovers to love disturbs the bond of love and, therefore, the bond's potential for lasting. The relationship itself becomes merely a bond of the past, to be remembered fondly perhaps, but not to be projected into the future. Because Ishtar has dissolved all of her past amorous bonds, Gilgamesh does not see any hope that he will fare any better with her. Her past establishes a pattern that Gilgamesh believes determines his future should he choose to take her up on her offer of love. Since love takes two consciousnesses with each consciousness playing the role of lover and beloved, Gilgamesh believes Ishtar's past failures are relevant when assessing her capacity for new love.

The idea behind a lasting love is that it survives the changes undergone by the lovers. So, as the hair grays, the kids grow, the jobs change, and even as society itself becomes unrecognizable in its new mores, technologies, and the like; the lovers will still love each other. A lasting love transcends change. But at what threshold of change is it acceptable to call off the love and consign it to the past tense rather than to look towards its indefinite future? Steady relationships in high school, seemingly on their way to blossoming into marriages, are often upset by the changes brought about by college life. One partner heads to a dorm, meets new people, learns new truths, and soon he or she "has changed" irrevocably. Everyone changes. This is not surprising, but in many cases, the changes brought about by college life render the partner less recognizable in interests, goals, and experiences. These changes may take one or both of the partners away from the bond, and love fades.

William Shakespeare proposed that "love is not love" at all if it falters under the pressures of change:

> Let me not to the marriage of true minds
> Admit impediments. Love is not love
> Which alters when it alteration finds,
> Or bends with the remover to remove:
> O, no! it is an ever-fixed mark,

That looks on tempests and is never shaken;
It is the star to every wandering bark,
Whose worth's unknown, although his height be taken.
Love's not Time's fool, though rosy lips and cheeks
Within his bending sickle's compass come;
Love alters not with his brief hours and weeks,
But bears it out even to the edge of doom.
If this be error and upon me proved,
I never writ, nor no man ever loved.[11]

Marriage is a proclamation that the lovers will not allow changes to interfere with their bond. Love "looks on tempests and is never shaken." In the traditional wedding vow, one promises "To have and to hold for richer or for poorer, in sickness and in health, all the days of my life, till death do us part." Of course, many marriages fail and we might observe, along with Shakespeare, that the apparent love was not *true* love ("Love is not love which alters when it alteration finds").

This thinking that a love that dies was never really love at all suffers from a major drawback, which we might classify as a falsifiability problem. How could we ever prove that Shakespeare was wrong about love, that love could be true even though it did not survive change? As soon as it ends, the "Shakespeares" would declare that it wasn't a real love. We could never prove the others wrong in their thinking that true love lasts. In short, "true love" contains the information that it "lasts" as much as "pentagon" contains the information that it has "five sides." If a figure was found that had less than five sides, it would not be a pentagon. If a relationship was found that did not last, it would not be true love. The logic of the problem definitely invites concerns, but nevertheless, the meaning of the traditional wedding vow does offer the hope for a love which always outpaces any changes in the circumstances of the lovers.

Of course, love might grow throughout the changes, not merely survive. This is the hope:

Those lines that I before have writ do lie,
Even those that said I could not love you dearer:
Yet then my judgment knew no reason why
My most full flame should afterwards burn clearer.
But reckoning Time, whose million'd accidents
Creep in 'twixt vows, and change decrees of kings,
Tan sacred beauty, blunt the sharp'st intents,
Divert strong minds to the course of altering things;
Alas! why, fearing of Time's tyranny,
Might I not then say, 'Now I love you best,'
When I was certain o'er incertainty,
Crowning the present, doubting of the rest?
Love is a babe, then might I not say so,
To give full growth to that which still doth grow?[12]

A love that grows is a fine example of unqualified love because of its promise to maintain itself into the indefinite future. A love that grows has a better chance to last than a love that merely survives. Whether love survives or grows, life on earth remains the context for lasting love. The wedding vow, recall, is until "death do us part." In other words, death (or, as Shakespeare writes in Sonnet CXVI, "the edge of doom") is the change, unlike going to college, that seemingly allows for the bond of love to be legitimately severed. When one lover loses his or her life, that lover is no longer present to the world in the same sense that other humans are present. At this point, the remaining lover grieves and misses his or her deceased beloved.

Yet many go on to find new spouses confident that they have remained faithful to previous vows. They are not Ishtars. How can this be when love implies the eternal and boundless? One response is that when the poets speak of "undying love" and "loving forever and a day," they may mean that the love is permanent as long as the lovers shall live. On this view, the undying love is not really undying: there is a disparity between what is said and what is meant. The love is undying only as long as the participants are alive. Without one or both participants, there is no relationship (broadly speaking). A narrower conception of a relationship may very well include two living humans who part company, separate geographically, and do not interact in any way except to share the same world. Such people would have, I would say, a non-interacting relationship. We have relationships with many people whom we refuse to acknowledge, but this does not eliminate the fact that there really is a relationship. If we can agree that a relationship involves two humans who are alive, then the end of the relationship would be logically prior to the end of a loving relationship. By this I mean that to have a loving relationship presupposes having a relationship. One cannot have a loving relationship without first having a relationship. But death ended the relationship. Without any relationship, there is *a fortiori* no love relationship and there is no non-love relationship. The love has never died, because the relationship didn't outlast the love. When the relationship outlasts the love, then we say that the love has died.

At the point in the story when Gilgamesh questions Ishtar which of her lovers she has loved forever, he knows she is an immortal goddess and he does not yet seem to realize that he will die. Gilgamesh's beloved friend Enkidu was still alive at the time and Gilgamesh did not understand the implications of his mortality. He did not understand that the gods established death without revealing its timing.[13] From what he understood at the time of Ishtar's proposal of love, he and Ishtar would continue to live indefinitely. So the upshot is that Gilgamesh still expected that Ishtar *could* love into the indefinite future and that she had developed the habit of not doing so.

But, for us, who are presumably privy to the lessons of mortality, what could the concept of "loving forever" mean? We do not know whether we will enjoy life at a later time, but we do know that we are living now. Loving forever has to do with loving into a tomorrow that has not yet unfolded. Loving forever gets its meaning from a trust that should a tomorrow be available (with all the changes it brings), both lovers will still be available to each other. For Ishtar and Gilgamesh (so he thought), every tomorrow would have been available. For us, we have good reason to hope that a tomorrow will indeed be available. Tomorrows usually are. In truth, only one day that we live does not have a tomorrow. Philosopher Blaise Pascal (1623–1662 CE) reminds us what the poets profess, that "Love has no age; it is always a child."[14] Shakespeare, in similar spirit, refers to love as a "babe." Of course, children and babies do not have many years behind them. They do, we assume here, have a bounty of years in front of them. Like the painter who spends less time and attention on a figure's index finger nail than on the figure's face, the lover is not attentive to the past, but to the future. Like the painted figure's index finger, the past is there and acknowledged. But it is overridden by care and attention to the future. For further example, consider athletic competitions and the past. It seems that the upcoming playoffs and championship are always more important than last year's playoffs and championship. This is, indeed, often true, especially for those athletes competing. Athletes and organizations are always competing against others and against history, although history in the form of records, statistics, and nostalgia cannot be overridden easily.

COMPARISON OF LOSSES AND THE SELF

We now have clearer notions of why we may hold fast to ideas of love eternal and what it means to be in love: to anticipate the continuation of the loving relationship into the indefinite future. We expect the other to "be there" and "be loving" if the other is able. The presupposition of indefinite existence that love makes, though, is so strong that the death of a lover shatters the one left behind. As philosopher Robert Olson writes:

> A man may be in love without having known suffering, if to be in love is to be infatuated or simply to be a faithful husband and father. But, in the former case what passes by the name of love is simply a nervous itch; in the latter case, a routine or habit. In its essence love is an attitude of care and concern for a being whose death or desertion is always possible and would be an irreparable personal loss.[15]

Love implies its continuation. This is why its ending is so distressing: love, which implies its continuation, does not continue. With our brandished notion of love, then, we could reply to a stoic like Epictetus (55–135 CE) who asks us to feel similarly for our own losses of beloved persons as we do about others' losses.[16] While the *general* features of the loss may be comparable (e.g., you and I both lose a spouse), the *specific* love relationship is not. My particular love involves a particular irreplaceable person and when the other is gone, my particular loss is rightly felt in a way that reflects the annihilation of *my* love expected to continue indefinitely. This analysis extends to self-love as well. Leo Tolstoy's (1828–1910 CE) Ivan Illych, quoted in the first chapter, cannot feel others' loss of life because he does not have the relation to other selves in the way that he relates to his own self.[17] He does not presuppose others' continued life to the significant extent he presupposes his own. Of course, Jesus admonishes this self-love, which implies the self's continuation, and says that if we truly desire our continuation, then we will have to paradoxically deny our self-interest in (at least earthly) continuation:

> Then he said to all, "If anyone wishes to come after me, he must deny himself and take up his cross daily and follow me. For whoever wishes to save his life will lose it, but whoever loses his life for my sake will save it."[18]

Ivan Illych and all the rest of us who cling to earthly life will find that we will get the opposite, like the driver in snow or sand who floors the gas pedal in order to get out of a small decline. But is it really a paradox to turn away from life in order to gain life? If the true interest is in a spiritual continuation, it is not really paradoxical to deny one's earthly self to achieve that spiritual continuation. If Christians recognized themselves as primarily spiritual beings, they would not cling to things on earth. The life gained by turning from the earth is a richer life. The wages for spiritual continuation is death to earthly self. This means that even the Christian who follows Jesus' demanding prescription has a self-love, which seeks the self's continuation in heaven. More will be said on the dualistic nature of humanity, soul and body, in the later chapters on spiritual immortality and earthly immortality.

At this time, I conclude that self-love is a form of love, which, among other preferences and desires, seeks the continuation of the self. An objection to this description of self-love is suicide. When one commits suicide, many would say that he loves himself too much and does not think seriously enough of those he leaves behind. However, what seems to be meant in such a case is that the suicidal person is too *selfish* to think of those left behind. He only thinks of his own escape. Being selfish is being overly self-centered; having little or no regard for others. Self-love is different. Having self-love is being appropriately concerned with one's well-being.

IMMORTALITY AND ITS CONSEQUENCES FOR LOVE

When humans settled down into agricultural villages beginning around 8000 BCE, their social evolution accelerated. Ideas concerning organization, language, knowledge, and spirituality were exchanged more quickly than ever before as the forces of necessity and community took hold. Individuality seems to have emerged later. John Hick (b. 1922 CE) speculates that it was not until around 800 to 200 BCE that human individuality becomes distinguishable from group identity.[19] Only when a concept of the autonomous self is recognized does a sharpened concept of personal immortality, living in a concrete and self-conscious sense beyond the grave, emerge. But with a concept of living forever in a self-conscious state, the concept of two persons loving each other forever begins to make sense. Persons may now transcend even death, since a death to this world is merely a change in the circumstance of self, more like moving to a new community than becoming nothing. The Mormons (Church of Latter Day Saints) are one of the few who maintain that marriages made on earth continue for eternity in heaven. They call this "sealing." (Of course, some Mormons prescribe polygamy and sealing, but this subject is best avoided for now.) If love is care, concern, and intimacy, maybe immortality aspirants should hope for love to continue forever, or at the very least, accept the possibility that it could go on and on and on and on. With a mixture of love as continued bonding into the indefinite future, it becomes conceivable that even death might not sever the bonds of love. The relationship persists even as it undergoes its most radical change imaginable. Perhaps a love that doesn't survive this ultimate change, this tempest, wasn't really love after all.

Of course, it may appear selfish for one's spouse to demand that his beloved is not to marry another should he die. But perhaps the spouse is wise to the truth of love rather than naïve and obstinately demanding. Perhaps he understands the implications that personal immortality has for lasting love: since the lovers continue to exist, albeit in different environments for a time, the love ought to be honored even for the time that the two are apart. Just as it is a violation of normative ethics to nurture a new relationship while the other is in a separate town, so it is unethical to nurture a new one while the other is living on in a separate realm. The lawful marriage vow may indeed mean "until *earthly* death do us part," but that does not imply that love necessarily ends. The law doesn't recognize that it continues because it does not have any interest in the matter, since laws are for earthlings! Few would concede that the laws we live under always correspond to metaphysical reality. Why must marriage law necessarily correspond to the "marriage of true minds"? The laws were designed for social purposes.

Fidelity in love even after the death of a spouse is demanded of women in the *Laws of Manu*, an early Hindu text expressing the oral traditions from over three millennia ago:

> A virtuous wife who after the death of her husband constantly remains chaste reaches heaven . . . But a woman, who from a desire to have offspring violates her duty towards her deceased husband, brings on herself disgrace in this world and loses her place with her husband in heaven . . . A faithful wife who desires to dwell after death with her husband must never do anything that might displease him who took her hand, whether he be alive or dead. At her pleasure let her emaciate her body by living on pure flowers, roots, and fruit but she must never even mention the name of another man after her husband has died.[20]

Children born to widows were not considered lawful by the ancient Indian State. The social pressure to follow these rules, which leaders surely claimed were designed with the intent to secure perpetual happiness between husband and wife, was strong and effective. It is likely that these laws aimed at maintaining a patriarchal order that was at odds with women's power to self-determination and, ultimately, at odds with women's happiness. The religious notion that the Hindu soul joins the totality of being and thus loses its individuality and self-consciousness upon *moksha* (release from the cycle of rebirths) would seem to make marriage in the afterlife practically difficult, since two selves cannot be disentangled from the rest. Nevertheless, this injunction against a widow seeking a new husband seems crafted not with wisdom of the divine order, but with the craftiness of a shrewd Critian politician.[21] The most basic tenets of Hinduism reject the idea that the self is preserved in differentiated form. So, to bring in afterlife rewards for this staying "true" to a deceased spouse has dubious Hindu theological justification.

LOVE AS A DISTRACTION FROM OUR MORTALITY

There are two major considerations for love as a distraction. The first is the religious consideration. Simply put, love for God and others takes the focus off of oneself and one's own earthly impermanence. Many religions have doctrines and prayers intended to help the faithful to self-deny. For some (but certainly not all) followers of religion, love for the divine and for fellow humans is so forcefully projected outward that they do not think about themselves. The self is lost in the contemplation of the other. There is a purpose to an individual life more lasting than the egoistic self. The self *serves* that purpose. St. Paul (d. 65 CE) tells the Corinthians that love "endures all things" and "never fails" (*1 Corinthians* 13:4–8). Ideally, one attached to the mission and practice of love forgets his own fragility and impermanence. St. Paul's words on love were intended for the religious who made God and the community of brethren the center of their thoughts and actions. Interestingly, these *Corinthians* words have become a mainstay reading at many Christian weddings. It has thus taken on romantic significance, professing the Shakespearean declaration that love remains steady throughout life's tempests. Love distracts us from our earthly finitude.

The second major consideration for love as a distraction has been pushed by the prolific filmmaker and author Woody Allen (b. 1935 CE). Through his many characters on the screen and in pages, Allen defends the standpoint that there is no afterlife and that the universe we inhabit is devoid of any general meaning. Without God and without a general meaning for the cosmos, humans have tended to find meaning in romantic love. We know that while we live, we will be carrying out daily activities juxtaposed by meaninglessness. We know we are going to die. We know that when we die, there is nothing. We love to distract ourselves from our inevitable, crushing and complete annihilation. From his film

September, two characters, Peter and Lloyd, express connections between impermanence, meaninglessness, and love:

> **Peter:** You feel so sure of that [meaninglessness of the universe] when you look out on a clear night like tonight and see all those millions of stars? That none of it matters?
>
> **Lloyd:** I think it's just as beautiful as you do, and vaguely evocative of some deep truth that always just keeps slipping away, but then my professional perspective overcomes me, a less wishful, more penetrating view of it, and I understand it for what it truly is: haphazard, morally neutral, and unimaginably violent.
>
> **Peter:** Look, we shouldn't have this conversation. I have to sleep alone tonight.[22]

The abruptly changing themes from Lloyd's lines and Peter's remark that they "shouldn't have this conversation" since he has no one to sleep with are not simply a comedic transition from the impersonal universe to the intimate bedroom. Contrast is good for humor, but the point is more profound. The loneliness the mortal human feels in the face of a cold and indifferent universe leads him to seek solace in others whether he knows the reasons for his erotic pursuit or not. Others' concerns become ours and our concerns become others', and we feel temporarily relieved of the burden of death and extinction when absorbed in the other. This relief can only be temporary since both lovers will die. Placing trust in the impermanent is bound to disappoint. But nevertheless, from Allen's perspective, a temporary distraction can be achieved. On the other hand, while the religious distraction expresses the absorption of the self into God, the religious distraction offers slightly more promise for actually achieving immortality through the absorption. This point is picked up again early in the last chapter of this book.

LOVE AS A REMINDER OF OUR MORTALITY

In an essay whose thesis is a few steps removed from the purpose of this book, Leon Kass (b. 1939 CE) makes the claim that human cloning would upset the natural order of human reproduction. One of the reasons to value and preserve that threatened natural order is that it inspires the virtues of selflessness and humility. As we find mates and create children with them, we admit our impermanence and thus, the procreative act can be seen as an act of humility. But more than an act of humility, it is an act of honesty. We implicitly acknowledge our certain death as we place more individuals into the world that will outlive us and who will one day, we hope, procreate more beings. Kass puts it thus:

The soul-elevating power of sexuality is, at bottom, rooted in its strange connection to mortality, which it simultaneously accepts and tries to overcome . . .
Sexuality . . . serves replacement; the two that come together to generate one
soon will die. Sexual desire in humans as in animals, thus serves an end that is
partially hidden from, and finally at odds with, the self-serving individual.
Whether we know it or not, when we are sexually active we are voting with our
own genitalia for our own demise. The salmon swimming upstream to spawn
and die tell the universal story: sex is bound up with death, to which it holds a
partial answer in procreation.[23]

If thought about correctly, then, love would not distract us from our self-interest,
which includes the powerful desire not-to-die. Love is a *reminder* that we will in
fact die and by loving, we admit our mortality. Both of the lovers implicitly acknowledge their replacement, a replacement necessitated by each lover's impermanence.

PRECLASSICAL GREEKS: MYTH AND THE AFTERLIFE : THE BIRTH OF EROS

Hesiod (c. 775 BCE) and Homer (c. 750 BCE) were the chief influences on
early Greek myth. Informed by their own inherited traditions, these two poets set
down explanations of the gods' origins and their interventions in human affairs.
Hesiod, in his *Theogony*, points out that Eros [Love] came along quite early in
the generation of the gods:

First of all, the Void (Chaos) came into being, next broad-bosomed Earth, the
solid and eternal home of all, and Eros [Desire], the most beautiful of the immortal gods, who in every man and every god softens the sinews and overpowers the prudent purpose of the mind.[24]

The Void, Earth, and Eros notably do not have their causal ancestry traced
back to their precise origins. It was certainly not uncommon to leave the ultimate origins of the gods undetermined. See, for instance, the "Creation Hymn"
of the Hindu *Rig Veda* (c. 1300 BCE). The *Rig Veda's* author admits that he
does not know where the gods, or creation for that matter, come from. For the
Greek Hesiod, even Earth, which is the "eternal" home of all, did not always
exist. It came into being: he is just vague on the details.

Hesiod refers to Eros as immortal, but Eros comes into being after the Void
and seemingly after Earth.[25] (Immortality for Hesiod is about future limitlessness and not about the past.) That Eros "softens the sinews and overpowers the
prudent purpose of the mind" has long been known. Its empirical proof is all
around. It breaks up families, and prods many to start them before they *think*
they are "ready," and even to start them with people with whom they are not
particularly well-matched. Hesiod portrayed Eros as unable to be controlled, and
his own contemporaries must have, like us, acknowledged its power. Even so,

Eros is to be welcomed and not to be feared, because, on balance, it is necessary. Some would say that Eros imparts immortality, because this god leads us to reproducing fresher members of our species. These members are causal links in the human chain leading into the indefinite future. As Plato (427–347 BCE) would later explore in his *Symposium*, Eros leads us into questions concerning the prospects for and desirability of physical species-immortality (progeny). Plato picks up on the notions of love and immortality to challenge whether progeny is the goal of true love and whether immortality by physical love is the best kind of immortality.

LOVE AND IMMORTALITY IN PLATO'S 'SYMPOSIUM'

The Athenian Plato wrote a series of dialogues in which his teacher Socrates engages in conversations about definitions, knowledge, and virtue. In the *Symposium* dialogue, Socrates (469–399 BCE) attends a drinking party where the guests converse about Eros, or love. Symposiums were common in Greek culture and were recognized forums for revelry and spirited discussion. Women were not allowed at these parties.

The discussion over love, in the *Symposium*, soon leads the men to consider beauty, posterity, fame, and Idealism. In the pages that follow, I shall present Socrates's case that (1) beauty is the mechanism which attracts love, that (2) the object of love is either material or immaterial and that (3) the lover of the immaterial pursues the Forms and that (4) the Soul's makeup is akin to the Forms. In the next chapter, on fame, I shall further explore Socrates's claim to those at the symposium that, normatively speaking, immortality through mental activity (pursuing the immaterial) is far superior to immortality through progeny and descendents (pursuing the material).

Eros implies attraction, and attraction implies that the attracted finds beauty in the attractive. Clearly Eros and beauty are intertwined. (Can we love somebody or something we do not think is beautiful in a compelling way?) The view of Eros that Socrates proposes he claims to have learned from a priestess named Diotima.[26] We begin with naïve notions of love, Socrates recounts, gleaned from individual experiences and ascend our way to true notions of beauty. One may, in a sense, measure love by the rubric of what is most beautiful. The lover ascents to true beauty by:

> climbing from the love of one person to love of two; from two to love of all
> physical beauty; from physical beauty to beauty in human behavior; thence to
> beauty in all subjects of study; from them he arrives finally at that branch of
> knowledge which studies nothing but ultimate beauty. Then at last he understands what true beauty is.[27]

Here we see in Diotima the Platonic hope to transcend this world where beautiful objects and beautiful people come to be and pass away, or in generalized terms, the people who may serve as impermanent objects of beauty.[28] So, in

Plato, we see reasserted the Pythagorean claim that the standard and form of ultimate reality is not dependent upon earthly expressions.[29] This view proposes, like all of Plato's Forms, that beauty "exists for all time, by itself and with itself" and it is "unique."[30] The lover has a choice of which world of beauty to live in: the material or the immaterial.

Diotima, Socrates, and Plato find the view outlined above especially appealing because the observable world of beauty offers too many examples of things partially beautiful, but not wholly so. That world offers too many examples of things once beautiful losing that beauty through aging and decay. It does not befit a wise person to indulge in the lesser and corruptible beauties such as "sexy people," for example, when he might otherwise contemplate the greatest and undying beauty, the Form of beauty itself.

This derision of material beauty is unsubtly returned to by Plato when Alcibiades enters the symposium and recounts a story when Socrates did not choose to indulge in sensual pleasure with the willing Alcibiades, proving that Socrates keeps his mind on immortal notions of beauty rather than on fleeting beauty. Alcibiades follows his passions, as shown in Jean-Baptiste Regnault's (1754–1829 CE) 18th century painting *Socrates Tears Alcibiades from the Embrace of Sensual Pleasure*, but Socrates sets his attentions on higher things. So, we get a rather forceful statement where human love ought to be directed: towards the permanent, towards the lasting. The final scene of the *Symposium* thus joins the *Apology*, *Crito*, and *Phaedo* to testify to Socrates's commitment to wisdom over bodily comfort, imprisonment, and pleasure.

If we love the immortal Forms, then we are in love with something that is close to the nature of the human soul. The soul is most at home with this love. Plato's doctrine of the Forms does indeed stake the Forms as immortal, not in the sense of godlike, but in a sense that the philosophers from Anaximander to Pythagoras anticipate: Immortal process and principle underpin our sensible experience.[31] Plato, in outlining his immortal Forms, offers arguments for the immortality of the soul in his account of Socrates's hour of death, the *Phaedo*. One important argument, from our perspective of love and immortality, compares the existence of an undying soul to the immaterial Forms:

> Then the soul is more like the invisible than the body; and the body is like the visible . . . Have we not also said that, when the soul employs the body in any inquiry, and makes use of sight or hearing, or any other sense — for inquiry with the body means inquiry of the sense — she is dragged away by it to the things which never remain the same, and wanders about blindly, and becomes confused and dizzy, like a drunken man, from dealing with things that are ever changing? . . . But when she investigates any question by herself, she goes away to the pure, and eternal, and immortal, and unchangeable, to which she is akin, and so she comes to be ever with it, as soon as she is by herself, and can be so; and then she rests from her wanderings and dwells with it unchangingly, for she is dealing with what is unchanging. And is not this state of the soul called wisdom?[32]

Notice that Plato makes the claim that the individual soul is "akin" to the "pure, eternal, immortal, and unchangeable." The term 'eternal,' for Plato, means that something always exists: Plato believed that the soul pre-exists the body. The term 'immortal' applies to the future, but not necessarily to the past: to be immortal, a being, which may not have existed at all points in the past, must never die. The focus is on the future life of the immortal.

For Plato, the study of love, which aims at true beauty, ultimately reveals the properties of the Forms and some of those properties are likened to the human soul: namely, the properties of immortality and immateriality. The *Symposium* view of love defended by Socrates as convincing is certainly more hopeful than the view of love as a temporary distraction from utter extinction expressed by Woody Allen's *September* characters. For Plato, a love absorbed in the permanent and transcendent is far superior to a love absorbed in the impermanent and immanent.

The concepts of permanent versus impermanent are important considerations for fame and whether fame-seeking is successful and worthwhile.

CHAPTER THREE: FAME

The best choose one above all else: everlasting fame above mortals. The majority are contented like well-fed cattle.—Heraclitus

Gentlemen, I entrust to you the most precious thing on earth, my fame.—Louis XIV

I shall now focus on fame as a way to attain immortality. To be famous involves being recognized and regarded as significant in the minds of others. Whereas the lover pursues love's continuation into the indefinite future, the fame-seeker pursues recognition and accolades into the indefinite future. In general, I shall examine and reexamine the issues of love and fame. I shall also take a more detailed look into the particular issues of what type of fame is best, the likelihood of fame, and the problem of infamy.

The relation between death and fame is of particular interest. One knows the reality of death approaches so one sets himself up, through deeds and demeanor, to be remembered beyond death. It is a mode of afterlife, or less euphemistically, of "afterdeath." For example, consider Jan Vermeer's (1632–1675 CE) *Art of Painting*, in which the death-signifying mask and the fame-signifying trumpet share the pictorial space through which the artist seeks to mark and extend the life of the woman by painting her. The painting may have just as aptly been called the *Art of Bestowing Fame*.

Death is the end of earthly life, but fame, if orchestrated well enough, might be counted on to carry on our influence. Vermeer may have connected death and fame in his painting, but Louis XIV, quoted in the preface to this chapter, made quite an effort to connect them on the canvas of the French political landscape. In his age of bold architecture, peerless sculpture, and golden age painting,

Louis XIV's artists were up to the challenge of drawing attention to their bene-
factor. Louis XIV's robust public relations aimed to petrify his memory into the
minds of posterity. Fame was said to be Louis's most precious goal.

FAME IN PLATO'S 'SYMPOSIUM'

Fame-seeking is one response to death. Love and fame are nicely linked in
Plato's *Symposium* and I shall take the *Symposium*'s lead to allow the issue of
love to lead us into a discussion of fame. In what follows, I shall look into claim
of Diotima that the object of love determines what kind of immortality one
might receive, or even if immortality is possible. If one loves the physical, then
physical descendents are his immortality. If one loves the mental or heroic, then
everlasting fame is his prize. I shall also explore and criticize the Socratic argument that fame-seeking is worthwhile because of what fame offers the soul: immortality.

Diotima, the learned priestess who instructs Socrates on love, claims that
those who value reproduction via the physical turn to women and imagine immortality will come through their children.[1] On the other hand, those who value
being remembered for all time will desire leaving behind an "undying memory"
from heroic undertakings. Some leave behind such a lasting memory by courage, such as the warrior Achilles, and others do it by mental creativity, such as
Homer.

Put into a disjunction of prescriptions, then, we have two choices: (1) we
ought to pursue biological immortality, or (2) we ought to pursue fame. The
second choice may be further subdivided into the following: (2a) to pursue fame
by acting courageously, or (2b) to pursue fame by using our mental creativity.

As for whether we ought to pursue biological immortality (1) or fame (2),
Diotima is clear that we ought to pursue fame (2). Diotima proposes that being
the object of "undying memory" is better than being an ancestor of the biological kind:

> We would all choose children of this kind for ourselves, rather than human
> children. We look with envy at Homer and Hesiod, and the other great poets,
> and the marvelous progeny they left behind, which have brought them undying
> fame and memory . . . They have published to the world a variety of noble
> achievements, and created goodness of every kind. There are shrines to such
> people in honor of their offspring, but none to the producers of ordinary chil-
> dren.[2]

It has been suggested that Diotima's implicit reasons for valuing fame over children is that fame preserves the individual whereas the children preserve, merely,
the species.[3]

Socrates, who is often remembered as *the* perennial doubter, accepts
Diotima's praise for fame. Of course, it is not surprising that Socrates accepts
this *Symposium* argument that devalues the physical. Socrates made a career out

of scorning the physical and celebrating the mental. However, on some level, even Socrates must concede that the physical acts of procreation make possible the remembrance of the mental acts of procreation. Just as Socrates would have to admit that the physically inclined, appetitive-type manual laborers of the *Republic* provide the leisure time for the Guardians to pursue their intellectual projects[4], it seems we'd have to admit that those men who "turn to women" (and women who "turn to men") reproduce the future generations who will visit the shrines and honor the famous achievers of days gone by. Without future generations, recognition and regard, or in short, fame, dissolves. To this Socrates could reply that the *necessity* of physical reproduction for fame does not entail that physical reproduction *is better* than fame, just as the physical necessity of sleep for waking life does not entail that sleep is better than waking life. We must examine in greater detail this question of necessity, but before doing so, let us look into the argument that prizes fame earned by mental accomplishment above fame earned by courageously achieved excellence.

OUGHT WE TO PURSUE FAME BY USING OUR MENTAL CREATIVITY?

What, then, is the best way to earn fame: fame earned by wisdom and knowledge, or fame earned by courage and honorable activity? Presuming that the individual seeks to immortalize himself by fame, we should consider why the individual may be better preserved by fame earned by wisdom and knowledge. Recalling that Homer earned his fame by wisdom and Achilles earned his fame by courage, we may begin to note why Homer seems better preserved than the courageous Achilles:

> What is preserved [of Achilles] is the persona, the mask. It is not Achilles. Thus, even if the begotten is good, if it is no more than this, it can hardly be seen as a very successful pursuit of immortality . . . Homer, on the other hand, survives not as content, but as the work itself . . . He is the 'poet' who selected which actions and which people would be preserved. Homer is the one who delineated their characters for all time to come.[5]

Homer makes possible the remembrance of Achilles. Nevertheless, as Achilles's dependence on Homer should be recognized, this alone does not justify that Homer's fame is better than Achilles's. Remember that something's being necessary does not entail that it is better. (The physical reproducers are necessary for the fame of others, but such does not entail that the physical reproducers are equal to or better than the famous others.) Rather than overstate the importance of necessity, then, we ought to focus on the mental contributions of the selective and reflective mind: Homer chooses which aspects of Achilles are salient. Thus, we are constrained in our interpretation of Achilles because the author has only chosen to give us only certain parcels of the totality that was the fearsome warrior. In fact, the courageous do not leave behind any legacy of valor if not for the intellectual documenting it, and such documentation must be of sufficient quality to warrant being preserved and read. Like an artist choosing which features to depict, focus on, or even what perspective from which to see them, the mental creator wields much power even compared to the courageous hero.

However, we could conceive that the courageous, like the wise, operate from some rational principles. They too select and reflect information. For instance, in Plato's *Republic*, Socrates claims that being brave is a "conviction about the sort of things that it is right to be afraid of—the conviction implanted by the education which the law-giver has established."[6] Socrates betrays an understanding of courage that has mental content (i.e., it is "implanted by . . . education"). Convictions are not merely feelings. They are not comprised solely of affective content: they are beliefs replete with information. Yet, even so, it may be that the education, promulgated by more rational superiors, implants the beliefs requisite for courageous conviction. For Socrates, the wise in the *Republic* set the agenda of education since the wise alone, presumably, have the ability to discern what is truly good for the entire commonwealth. In the *Republic*, Socrates defends a social order that has the intellectuals ruling over the courageous:

> So, if a state is constituted on natural principles, the wisdom it possesses as a whole will be due to the knowledge residing in the smallest part, the one which takes the lead and governs the rest [the Auxiliaries motivated by courage and the tradesmen motivated by appetites].[7]

I believe these *Republic* insights support the *Symposium* view that rational persons (those contemplating the Forms and who love the mental) are in a better position compared to those who depend on the rational persons for guidance and direction. These *Republic* insights that the mental ruler *should* have significant control over the courageous runs parallel to the point that the mental creator has the power to make us remember, or in other words, to bestow fame onto the courageous. If one earns fame by mental creativity, that individual is preserved in his work. Actions of battlefield courage, whether documented or undocumented, evaporate into the past as all actions do. Mental contributions, however, under normal circumstances of documentation, are not subject to such a steep and abrupt diminution to nothingness. So long as they are mental *contributions* and not merely mental thoughts, they have far a better chance than actions to prevail against the time's evaporative power.

WHO BESTOWS FAME?

The power of the author to create memory has been harnessed by others since Homer. Some poets through the ages have made no apologies that they possessed the power to bestow undying fame. The Hellenist Theocritus (c. 3rd century BCE), for example, appealed to a Syracusan king for a court position. He tantalized the king with the proposition of fame. By poetry, he wrote the king:

You shall be rewarded when death hides you,
Not loiter by cold Acheron[8], shorn of your fame,
No better than a poor laborer with calloused hands . . .
Though living men make free with a dead man's goods,
The Muses' gift of fame can never be taken.[9]

Theocritus proposes that the fame he grants has power over death. Fame cannot be taken away like material possessions. Fame is attached to the individual. Material goods can change ownership quite readily. Money, a bicycle, books, a car, can belong to someone else. Fame is not transferable. Death severs our connections to things, but death cannot sever fame.

Shakespeare likewise thought that his poetry bestows fame, fame not to a king, prince, duke, or president: but rather, fame to a beloved:

Your monument shall be my gentle verse,
Which eyes not yet created shall o'er-read;
And tongues to be, your being shall rehearse,
When all the breathers of this world are dead;
You still shall live, such virtue hath my pen.[10]

Perhaps astonishingly, Shakespeare believes so strongly in the power of his words that he surmises his beloved "shall live" on even without anyone reading or reciting the poem ("When all the breathers of this world are dead"). Who has ever heard of fame without anyone alive to remember? This is remarkable. One wonders what Shakespeare would say if the words themselves were destroyed. It is likely that he would say that his ideas, expressed by his words, are undying: such virtue hath his mind!

In the case of all three poets, each poet chose whether to write or not to write about the persons and deeds involved. Homer's Achilles, Theocritus's Syracusan king, and the beloved in the Shakespeare sonnet could each claim that without his or her inspiration there would be no poems. True enough, those referred to in the poems could argue that it is they and their deeds which call out for someone to take time and expend talent to write about them. However, isn't it more likely that the creative writers would have simply chosen other persons and deeds to write about? There are a lot of extraordinary people on contemporary streets, and many more who walked the streets of the past. The mental creator is free to choose and reject in a way that the dependent courageous person is not. Many heroes have never been put on pedestals.

The great Florentine painter Sandro Botticelli (1445–1510 CE) provides an analogue to the poets who acknowledge themselves as fame givers. His *Adoration of the Magi* painting is a distinctly Renaissance attempt to bring religious events into the present, giving them a new relevance for his patrons. Yet the pandering to the Medicis' sense of their own desert and superiority is so very evident. The patriarch of the wealthy commissioning family, Cosimo de' Medici (1389–1464 CE), kneels down before the baby Jesus and the Virgin Mary. The ruins in the immediate and receding background signal connections to, yet departures from, the grandeurs of the Roman past. The worlds of Christianity of ancient Rome comfortably coexist. The worlds of the past, with its ruins and Christian figures, and the present, with its self-confident and successful merchant prima donnas are at home with one another. Truly, to pull of these seemingly competing iconographies with such grace and formal technique is a feat of Botticelli's mental creativity.

Surely Diotima and Socrates would herald Botticelli's work. Yet further inspection of the painting also reveals a self-conscious attempt to ensure the individual fames of artist and patrons alike. Botticelli's likeness glances out from the painting's lower left corner. Most of the figures are recognizably members of the Medici inner-circle. The religious significance of the well-to-do bowing down before the Christ becomes lost in their fine clothes and intriguing asides. Who is *really* glorified in the painting?[11] Botticelli's "mental creativity" may in fact be a symptom of fame-seeking rather than virtue.

Botticelli's gifts of fame to himself and to the Medicis should make us question whether any fame accrued as a result of the painting is tainted because it was so ostentatiously sought. It seems, to most of us anyway, that we do not want to "award" someone with fame if they so blatantly seek it. Yet for Diotima, the drive for earned fame prompts us to perform excellent acts and leave behind enduring legacies and artifacts of value. To the priestess, the drive for fame is valuable in itself. Far from a distraction, the desire for fame is a catalyst for individuals to do excellent things.[12] As Francis Bacon (1561–1626 CE) put it, "Fame is of that force, as there is scarcely any great action, wherein it hath not a great part."[13] Botticelli's painting is well-recognized as fine art, which has a distinct creativity, and, therefore, seems worthy in itself and independent of its painter's motivations.[14] We would do well to honor its worth regardless of the spurious intentions of its creator.

Diotima's argument, that the mental virtues are superior to courageous ones, persuades Socrates. Diotima and Socrates are at odds with the views of their Greek contemporaries who saw the warrior equipped with courage as the finest possible individual and, therefore, the best candidate for deserved fame. The sculpture of the *Aegina Warrior* (c. 500 BCE), for instance, and the laudable epic poem *Iliad* (c. 800 BCE) illustrate the centricity of courage in civic life. But now, according to Diotima, what is left behind by the courageous is outshined by what is left behind by the intellectual. Even by the time of Socrates (469–399 BCE), most Athenians probably weren't ready to demote the status of courage in favor of the mental. After all, did the intellectuals defeat the Persian invaders?[15] Did the intellectuals build the economic machine that produced, transported, and imported goods from all over the Mediterranean? Intellectuals are frequently caricatured as thinkers and not doers. They are questioners without answers. And, weren't the intellectuals responsible for the softening of faith in Athenian values, and hence, Athens' military loss against Sparta? Many

Athenians blamed the pesky Socrates for the loss against Sparta in 404 BCE. He insubordinately challenged the Athenian leaders and corrupted the resolve of the next generation, they thought. He was a man of inaction in a world that needed the opposite.[16] Most Greeks in those days must have thought it laughable if not dangerous to claim that soldiers such as Achilles were inferior to thinkers like Socrates.

WHAT IS PRESERVED BY FAME?

Just *what* is preserved in the written word of the writer and subject is a matter for reflection and debate. Certainly, it is not the personality of the famous that is preserved. Homer does not live merely because we think about him and his work. Is it the objects valued by the deceased? Horace (65–8 BCE) announces that those valuables are squandered by the living: "After your death, the lavish heir will quickly drive away his woe; the wine you kept with so much care along the marble floor shall flow."[17] What is preserved of the mental creativity? How long can the artifacts of mental creativity last? Ideally, they can last indefinitely. But statues break and walls crumble. Paper is very susceptible to destruction. Only one piece of the Classical Greek musical repertoire remains.[18] One papyrus page, less than 40 notes, remains from the classical Greeks, who made theatre and music centerpieces of their civic and cultural lives. Sometimes the famous work itself, or the masterpiece of a famous person, does not survive.[19]

Returning to the remnant Greek music, a piece from *Orestes,* how could something so central to civilized life not have been preserved for the future? Common sense has one answer. The written word is actually less durable than most other creations because the mediums used to hold the words are fragile at best. More durable artifacts have been destroyed as well. Search Berlin for Heinrich Schliemann's Mycenaean discoveries (including pottery), and one learns what war can do to cultural artifacts. Go to Assisi and you'll find a veritable art museum-basilica suffered the devastation of a 1997 earthquake. Cambodia's *Angkor Wat* is the largest religious complex of the ancient world (it contains treasures of Buddhist art), yet its long bas relief friezes are wearing away with the extremes of moisture and aridness, which characterize the region's weather patterns. Moreover, preservationists struggle not only with wars, disasters, and nature itself, they struggle also with the transience of the painters' paints as well as the author's ink (see, for example, the Vatican preservationists' attempts to preserve their archives which include one of the last surviving letters in the pen of Michelangelo). It is understandable, given the fragility of tangible material, that a particularly vulnerable material such as written music cannot be trusted in itself to survive long enough to bring eternal fame. Computers and digital preservation may temper the risk of certain artifacts becoming completely obsolete, but they also exacerbate the likelihood that important correspondences will be lost. Delete. That's it. *What* is preserved depends on circumstances far beyond the control of the fame-seeker.

Just *where* it is preserved (on the paper, in the computer coding, in God's mind, in progeny's mind) is even more contentious. Leonardo Da Vinci's (1452–1519 CE) *Last Supper* is in sorry shape and prints of it may actually express the essence of the work better than the original. The real painting is not what most believe it to be. The real painting's suggested image is more famous than the true image. Marcel Duchamp's (1887–1968 CE) *Fountain* exists only in replica form (materially speaking), but its conceptual form (the idea) inspires and challenges us to broaden our conceptions of art. It is famous.

Phidias's (c. 480–430 BCE) *Parthenon Athena* has been lost, but it is famous. Posterity recognizes the mental achievements of Da Vinci, Duchamp, and Phidias even if, respectively, the material legacy is compromised, a copy, or lost. These creators have taught us to see the world differently whether in terms of religion and emotions, modern life and assembly-line economies, or civic self-image and religious guardianship. Yet much of their output is assessed in our minds and supplemented by our minds, such that the original work is quite different from the remembered image. The remembered person, therefore, may be famous for doing something or for being someone that was quite separable from what he did or who he was in reality.

FAME MAY BE OVERRATED

Fame may be overrated and overstated. Fame may be wrongly predicated. One could argue that the creator of what is "left behind" does not really deserve the credit after all. Psychoanalyst Otto Rank (1884–1939 CE) argues that the posterity who bestows renown only does so to identify a general trend, not to create and nurture the personal memory of the famous. He concludes art to be "unintelligible without a consideration of its effect on its contemporaries and posterity — meaning thereby not its aesthetic but its social and cultural effect."[20] So, those truly responsible for fame are not the Homers, the Theocrituses, the Shakespeares, and the Botticellis. The responsible ones are the contemporaries who interpret culture rather than the creators who produce the work for interpretation. The fame-seeker can do very little to secure fame without the help of others. It is true, we must agree, that fame is dependent on others. We cannot force others to remember us and to give us proper credit. However, can't we also agree that one can take certain steps to better the chances for fame? Louis XIV (1638–1715 CE) could use his ministers, his subjects, and his wealth to saturate Europe with his image and commission great art to bring posterity to his palaces. To achieve renown and cultivate fame would presumably have been easier for Louis XIV than it will be for most of us. But even as the agent can take steps to increase the probability of fame, he cannot guarantee it. When Louis XIV died of gangrene in the grand palace at Versailles, he could only really *hope* the memory of him would remain forever vibrant. Into the hands of those capable of remembering him he commended his spirit.

THE CHANCES FOR IMMORTALITY THROUGH FAME

The Roman Emperor and philosopher-king Marcus Aurelius (121–180 CE) identified fame as vain and fame-seeking as unproductive when he wrote that:

> All things fade and quickly become legend, soon to be lost in total forgetting. This I say of those who shone in wondrous glory; as for other men, they are no sooner dead than "unknown, unheard of." But in any case, what is eternal remembrance? It is altogether vain…All is ephemeral, the one remembering and the one remembered.[21]

Aurelius is striking in his denial of Diotima's claim that fame and fame-seeking are worthwhile and good. Aurelius, who quotes the Greek philosopher Heraclitus (c. 535–475 BCE) elsewhere in his *Meditations*, clearly does not believe in the Heraclitean aphorism that "the best choose fame above all else."

The writer of the Biblical *Ecclesiastes*, too, philosophizes[22] that

> No one remembers what has happened in the past, and no one in days to come will remember what happens between now and then . . . No one remembers wise men and no one remembers fools. In days to come, we all will be forgotten.[23]

There seems to be something to the *Meditations* and the *Ecclesiastes* claims that eternal remembrance is vain and impossible. Assuming the human race will continue forever, we will likely be less remembered as the generations proceed from the point of our death. Even the Catholic Saints far outnumber those acknowledged by most Catholics. If Catholics don't remember them, who will? Olympic records change hands forever leaving the former record holders moving down long lists and off of short lists. How many of the almost seven billion humans on earth ever think of Khufu? — He presided over the building of a wonder of the world.

The more people that live, the more deceased, once-famous people will be forgotten. Homer and Hesiod had been dead only 400 years when the *Symposium* Diotima had declared them to possess "undying fame and memory." Granted that Homer is still reasonably well-known, Hesiod is less known, and the Spartan Lycurgus (c. 750 BCE) also mentioned by Diotima is hardly famous now. Perhaps Diotima's declaration was premature. One would need to be immortal to be certain that his own, or anyone else's, fame is "undying." This question may be asked of any famous person: what effect will an additional one-thousand years of human accomplishment have on his fame?

But suppose the famous could remain in the collective consciousness forever even amidst the ever-increasing competition for a place in it. Suppose fame were possible. *Should* we be concerned with how we will be remembered? Wouldn't our energies be better exerted on other matters?[24] As mentioned, Diotima thinks that we should be concerned with how well we will be thought of, since this concern prompts superior performance in those other matters. One could, of course, become so obsessed with how he will be thought of by posterity that he neglects the present and leads an inactive and forgettable life.

But alas, the sad fact is that the human race is likely not to survive forever. The last person with the knowledge of people and deeds (the last "one remembering" as Marcus Aurelius puts it) will die. Our expanding universe will suffer what physicists refer to as a 'heat death.' In the far-off future, the universe will cease to offer enough energy for sustainable human life. Another unforeseen natural cataclysm may finish us off before then. Perhaps we'll even kill *ourselves* off. We don't know for sure how or if the end will come about, but no informed thinker denies that it probably will. We must at least try, along with Shakespeare, to conceptualize a time "when all the breathers of this world are dead." Famous people will become an empty set. No one will remember them because no one will be alive. Someone who no one remembers is not famous. Everyone will be a someone who no one remembers. Therefore, the pursuit of undying fame belongs in the set of futile activities. The works themselves will not survive either. Even of the towering figure Plato, Leo Strauss observes: "Some day not a single copy of Plato will exist, which shows that if we put our trust in culture or civilization we are not very wise."[25]

The reproducer of people is, for Diotima, on the wrong side of immortality, since all people die. The reproducer of mental creativity is, for Diotima, on the right side of immortality, since undying recognition continues. Yet as we have seen, fame itself could not survive the death of the human race. The continuance of the human race and its principal methods of physical reproduction are the only guarantors that the famous will continue to be recognized. Fame may sometimes have a longer lifespan than the average human being, but it also must, in the end, be recognized as mortal.

WHAT SOCRATES SHOULD HAVE FOUND CONVINCING

If we review the Forms for a moment, we remind ourselves of the type of true immortality that Socrates found the most worthwhile. The Forms are invisible, unchanging, eternal, immortal, and pure.[26] Socrates specifically argues in the *Phaedo* that the soul is most akin to the Forms rather than the body and, therefore, we should seek the Forms rather than the body, which is frequently deluded by the physical world.[27] On this point, Socrates is perfectly consistent in accepting Diotima's arguments that discourage attention to the physical, exemplified by her following hypothetical:

> Suppose it were granted to someone to see beauty itself quite clearly, in its pure, undiluted form — not clogged up with human flesh and coloring, and a whole lot of other worthless and corruptible matter. Now, imagine he were able

to see the divine beauty in its own unique essence. Don't you think he would find it a wonderful way to live, looking at it, contemplating it as it should be contemplated, and spending his time in its company?[28]

However, Socrates' implicit rationale for wholeheartedly accepting the argument cited above is that the soul is akin to the incorruptible and eternal Form of beauty.[29] Yet Diotima's rationale does not include the proposition that humans at their core are like (or "akin" to) the divine object. On the contrary, her lack of faith that the soul is like the divine object in terms of its potential immortality is clear: "What is mortal tries to the best of its ability to be everlasting and immortal. It does this in the only way it can, by always leaving behind a successor to replace what decays."[30] And William S. Cobb emphasizes Diotima's denial of the immortal human:

> The denial of human immortality seems to be repeated at the end of Diotima's remarks when she says that the person who gives birth to true virtue will 'become a friend of the gods, and if any human being could become immortal, he would' (*Symposium* 212a) — the implication being that the hypothetical possibility cannot be fulfilled.[31]

The upshot is that Socrates and Diotima accept the same ascending hierarchy of the love of body, love of mind, and love of Forms for significantly different reasons. Their different rationales regarding the Forms and their relation to the human soul sheds light on the truly Socratic rationale for celebrating fame over children. Whereas Socrates' reason is that the soul is drawn towards the Forms because it shares characteristics with them, Diotima's reason is that the soul nobly attempts to be what it cannot really be: immortal. The inconsistency of rationales presents a major problem for scholars who would like to maintain that Diotima is Plato's mouthpiece in the *Symposium*. But even those who reject the Diotima–Plato connection behold that same problem when they hear Socrates tell the gallery at the party that he finds the account convincing.[32] Let us try to extract some additional considerations about Diotima's account before looking into more identifiably Socratic solutions on why fame is worth pursuing.

As we have already examined, fame will not last if there are no minds to contemplate the famous. Without human immortality, there are no minds to contemplate the famous. Diotima contends that the pursuit of fame is (1) nobler than begetting children (because fame emphasizes the mental over the physical) and (2) more successful than begetting children (presumably, because it usually outlasts bloodlines). But she endorses fame most of all because it is the best overall option for immortality: "This, Socrates, is the mechanism by which mortal creatures can taste immortality."[33] But if fame is known to be temporary, then the best option is not good enough. Immortality is not tasted at all: the only thing tasted is the *deception* that immortality is assured.

Daniel Anderson interprets Diotima as suggesting that immortality is indeed tasted, but only insofar as the *processes* of physical reproduction, fame, and creation are eternal.[34] We participate in processes greater than ourselves. If correct, Anderson's straightforward interpretation nevertheless invites a few interesting questions. First, why should Diotima value the fame of the individual more than the continuation of the species when the process of sex and birth for all members of the human species is likely to far outlast any one particular individual's renown? Secondly, we have an explanation problem: how is it that the creators of pyramids, mausoleums, poetry, and the like, are better understood as participants in a process rather than self-conscious curators and preservationists of their individuality? Is this the best explanation for Shakespeare, Botticelli, and Khufu? It certainly seems that they consciously aspired for individualized fame. Thirdly, why shouldn't individual achievement, such as Homer's, be the proper object of remembrance rather than the process of creation itself?

Beyond these questions, there is a practical problem to achieving lasting fame. Indeed, it is probably true that we all desire to have our good deeds live on after we die. However, many of us will also acknowledge the difficulty in attaining prolonged fame, especially when compared to the relative ease with which we can attain new children! The likelihood for the vast majority of us is that our great grandchildren will barely think of us. So, even those who would most likely pay our memories heed, will not. The very fact that they will exist to ignore us supports the supposition that physical reproduction is overwhelmingly a more dependable means of tasting immortality.

It seems that once we take personal immortality off the table (roughly, either the kind of vigorous spiritual immortality associated with the major western religions or the kind of extended life on earth that prolongevitists hope to bring about), then the main goal is to have *some part* of our lives live on. If *some part* is what's important, then physical reproduction seems more up to the task. But Socrates could still concede the fact that physical reproduction is somewhat effective (and even necessary as we have noted earlier), but nevertheless continue to maintain that physical reproduction is NOT the *noblest path* to immortality. However, for Socrates to make this claim, he would need to supplant Diotima's lack of faith in personal immortality with something more Socratic.

In the *Apology*, Socrates entertains the following disjunction concerning death: we either shall endure a total and irretrievable loss of consciousness upon the body's death, or, upon death, we shall journey to another place to continue living.[35] Now, if death were an irretrievable loss of total consciousness, Socrates would be susceptible to two earlier considerations that fame runs out eventually. First, the collective human memory constantly reorganizes and replaces the famous, and secondly, the collective human memory will someday cease altogether. The total loss of consciousness that death brings would be the death knell of fame. We are then left to wonder how Socrates can support fame as a better route than children when seeking immortality: fame is really no route at all.

The option besides loss of total consciousness presents its own problems. Suppose we journey to another place to continue living, then Socrates would retain his personality and, as he understands it, his proclivity to questioning those around him. Socrates says that he would die repeatedly if such were the case, since he would remain himself with his personality and memories intact. [36] Socrates thus rejects the Homeric conception, popular in his own day, that the surviving soul is but a shadow of its former self. If personal immortality were true, then even as the human beings eventually die out, human souls could continue living. Retaining their personal vitality and defining traits, humans could indeed persist with their memories of the famous. The afterlife would be full of rememberers.

With the addition of the personal immortality hoped for in the *Apology*, and supported in the *Phaedo*, we can make[37] the *Symposium* Socrates accept an argument about the priority of fame over children that he can defend using speculations from other dialogues: fame is a worthwhile pursuit because someone will always remember. Someone will always remember because someone will always live forever with his memories intact. Fame will therefore outlast physical reproduction. Yet this move invites a new problem, which is that no being desires what it already has, a point Socrates makes against Agathon in the *Symposium*. Socrates accepts that the fame-seeker desires immortality. But once we supplement this desire for the immortality of the soul with the claim that the soul is already immortal, the result is that some immortals (mortals with immortal souls) desire what they do not lack. To desire what one does not lack is impossible for Socrates:

> **Socrates:** Consider this proposition: anything which desires something desires what it does not have, and it only desires when it is lacking something. This proposition seems to me to be absolutely certain. How does it strike you?
>
> **Agathon:** Yes, it seems certain to me too.[38]

Of course, Socrates could avoid being trapped by his own words. First, he could argue that the immortality desired is properly understood as a quality of the Form of Beauty, rather than as a quality of his individual soul. True, the immortality of the soul is a precondition for permanently contemplating the eternal Form, but immortality is not the desire of the soul. So, at the deepest level, love remains a desire for what it lacks (and always will lack): the immortality and goodness *of the Form*. The *Phaedo* proposal is that the soul desires not its own qualities, but rather to behold knowledge: "Verily we have learned that if we are to have any pure knowledge at all, we must be freed from the body; the soul by herself must behold things as they are."[39] Perhaps after death, the soul that beholds the Forms would desire to behold them at a future time as well. Such a desire would, of course, be consistent with Socrates' notion that one's possessing something and desiring it at the same time essentially means that one desires to possess it at a future time.[40] It desires what it does not have *yet*—namely, future possession.

The fact that Socrates "finds convincing" Diotima's underdeveloped argument celebrating fame, which diverges from Socrates' thoughts about immortality expressed elsewhere, should move us to consider alternatives of interpretation on the intellectual rigor of Socrates, the efficacy of pursuing fame, and the connections between immortality and love. My own thoughts should be clear: because the Socrates of other dialogues saves Diotima's celebration of fame only by accepting the fundamentally different rationale of spiritual immortality, Socrates should not have been convinced by her initial argument, even though he agreed with the conclusion. An argument is comprised of premises and a conclusion. Good arguments are those in which the premises support the conclusion. It is indeed peculiar that the careful, ever-skeptical Socrates would have been so enamored by Diotima's acceptance of the Platonic hierarchy of body, mind, and Forms that he doesn't seem to notice her dispatching with the Platonic principles of the human soul. It is these principles that save, yet transform, the argument prioritizing fame over children into the new one Socrates should have found convincing. At this point, we have to continue to ask ourselves whether fame is a useful and trustworthy variety of immortality to pursue. To me, it seems that it is inextricably tied to the thesis of personal immortality and cannot stand on its own. Even so, we would be remiss to deny its power to lure our imaginations, attentions, and energies.

PREDICATING FAME OF SUBJECTS

How is fame ascribed? Certainly, we may grant fame to one who does not deserve it. Unfortunately for him, Richard Jewell (1962–2007 CE) was specified by media outlets and others as the Olympic bomber at the 1996 Atlanta games. Actually, Jewell (a private security guard) first alerted police of a suspicious package. He was a hero wrongly accused of being the villain. When Jewell died over ten years later, his obituaries (running across the nation) still identified him as the man falsely accused of the bombing. So, even after the truth came out, Jewell retained his fame. In truth, Eric Rudolph (b. 1966 CE) was the bomber. It would take the authorities some years to capture Rudolph and charge him, and it seems that Rudolph is more famous for eluding authorities than for the Centennial Olympic Park bombing itself.

One could miss out on deserved fame. The *Roettgen Pieta*'s (c. 1300 CE) sculptor (or sculptors) certainly deserves to be recognized for the statue's beauty. As many medieval sculptors and artists did, the sculptor worked not for credit (or even reference), but for the glory of God and the service of the Church.

One could become famous for base acts such as Herostratus's burning down the Temple of Artemis or John Wayne Gacy, Jr.'s murdering of innocent young men. We refer to this fame by the term 'infamy.' Do these scornful individuals deserve to be known more so than the Temple of Artemis's architects or Gacy's victims? The infamous are, in these cases, remembered better probably because their acts led to significant changes. Even if the changes are generally agreed be a worse state of affairs, the changes themselves draw our attention. This "drawing of our attention" is the shared characteristic of the famous and infamous.

There is no necessary connection between fame and virtue. Put another way, fame is value neutral. Saints sometimes go unnoticed. Heroes are sometimes remembered for the opposite things. Al Capone is famous and was probably not, on the whole, a virtuous man. When we talk about fame as a desire for a certain kind of immortality, though, we recognize that most do not seek fame earned by notoriety. Why not pursue notoriety? We seek fame to achieve immortality. The immortality we hope for, we think, should correspond with our self image.

Most of us do not consider ourselves arsonists, so we would not burn down George Washington's (1732–1799 CE) Virginian estate or throw the remaining papyrus from Euripides's *Orestes* score into a raging fire. Most do not seek attention through mass murder or assassination. Most of us think of ourselves as morally superior to killers, so that option of achieving fame is off the table *for us*. We do not open up ourselves to acquiring a fame that does not harmonize with our self image.

Notoriety can still creep in despite our best efforts. One might join a theatre production and have all the nights spent reciting and rehearsing culminate in botched lines and forgotten cues. Sports players who train hard and play well, most of the time, may attract notoriety for making one mistake. Worse, the negative fame may outshine and taint the many moments of accomplishment, as it did for Red Sox first-baseman Bill Buckner after he misplayed a ground ball in game six of the 1986 World Series. That the virtuous and notorious can each achieve fame only poses a consideration for those indifferent to all else but renown itself. Those who aim at fame to live on indefinitely desire that their fame and their identity match. Thus, Robert Nozick (1938–2002 CE) is correct to point out:

> The kind of trace one wants to leave is one that people know of in particular and that they know is due to you, one due (people know) to some action, choice, plan of yours, that expresses something you take to be important about the kind of person you are, such that people respect or positively evaluate both the trace and that aspect of yourself.[41]

One can be famous to his contemporaries and not-famous to posterity. Or, it could be the other way around, as the folk-musician Nick Drake's (1948–1974 CE) emerging legacy attests. In fact, the poet Petrarch (1304–1374 CE) expressed a possible reason for posthumous fame rather than fame enjoyed in one's life when he wrote, "Jealousy lives and dies with the body." And so, Petrarch continues, "The favor of humanity begins with the author's decease; the end of life is the beginning of glory."[42] Francis Bacon (1561–1626 CE) would later agree, adding that death "openeth the gate to good fame, and extinguisheth envy."[43] For Petrarch, seeking posthumous fame would be irrational for those who love life above all things, inasmuch as fame only comes about after death.

In this age of celebrity (I am not sure that it's an age of fame), people achieve renown in their own lifetimes. The media and the internet make it possible to be well-known within moments. Moreover, people become all-the-more recognizable through having their image and work countlessly repeated, or "looped." Nevertheless, mere fame as a variety of immortality fails for the subject seeking it, because without an afterlife, fame is not enjoyed by that subject. Again, fame is not enjoyed by the subject unless the subject has personal immortality. Perhaps Marcus Aurelius was correct to ask "What is it to you?" whether you achieve posthumous fame? If fame is the best future we have upon death, there is no "you" either to enjoy your fame (or to lament your dissolution into oblivion).

Fame can come to all sorts of things: animals, extinct animals, monuments, former monuments, past events, future events, living people, deceased people. Fame has to do with memory and consciousness. Those who are forgotten and left out of others' consciousnesses are not famous. Something may be famous for being what it is (e.g., the Grand Canyon, the son of Prince Charles) and it also may be famous for doing something (e.g., the author of *Being and Nothingness*, the tiebreaking judge in a landmark case).

Artists usually achieve their first fruits of fame by doing something creative. Their personality can then be sorted out from their work and, eventually, taken seriously. Andy Warhol (1928–1987 CE), the pop artist, became just as famous as his greatest works. The enigmatic yet introverted artist would command its own attention. This is not new, however, to art. Giorgio Vasari (1511–1574 CE), the first great art historian, wrote the *Lives of the Great Artists*, which made the artists famous in personality as well in work. The next chapter, on creative legacy, will look at the relations between creator, product, personality, and immortality. To be sure, we have already examined much on mental creativity and fame, but we shall now take an earnest look at mental creativity as a vehicle to leave behind lasting objects and ideas that will signal the continued presence of the creator on earth, even once he has left it.

CHAPTER FOUR: CREATIVITY AND LEGACY

No thought is born in me that has not "death" engraved upon it.—Michelangelo

The creative impulse in the artist, springing from his tendency to immortalize himself, is so powerful that he is always seeking to protect himself against transient experience, which eats up his ego.—Otto Rank

Some of us create children. Some of us create beautiful wood sculptures. The created person or sculpture did not exist at a previous time, but comes into being some time after its creator creates it. The creation is contingent, or in another term, dependent, upon its creator. There are many types of creative persons. There can be creative artists, creative intellectuals, creative statesmen, creative religious leaders, creative preschoolers, and so on. In this chapter, I shall examine some connections between creations and the creators' pursuits of immortality. After explaining how creations are parcels from the past that stand to influence the future, I shall look into the hopes of creators to have their creations *stand for them* into the as-yet-unfolded future, even after they depart this world. I shall go on to examine how the creator brings into being something both new and valuable. The creator thinks that the creation is new and valuable, and exists as his proxy. The creations themselves, since they are dependent upon their creators, give the creators lasting existence since a creation explicitly or implicitly references its creator. (That wheat field in front of you is the work of Van Gogh. That group portrait was painted by Rembrandt. Who composed this? — Oh, that piece is by Claude Debussy.)

The creative act need not result in an original, tangible object that persists into the future for the consequences of the creative act and, by reference, the creative person to live on. An example that comes quickly to mind is the conceptual artists, whose ideas are primary. Of course, concepts must be codified into some form (e.g., language or structured presentation) to be expressed and communicated, but the creation itself does not need to remain in its original form as such. Duchamp's "original" *Fountain* is lost, but this doesn't matter (at least is does not matter to the art history textbook editors and art auction participants who, respectively, print the replica and buy it at auction). Similarly, the German artists with head lice who lived in an Israeli museum to explore the analogy of "host" and (unwelcomed) "guest" left behind no tangible object.[1]

THE PAST

Creations by definition reach a certain threshold of completed-ness, which situates them as items in the "past." Yet, these contributions have extended life and potential influence into the indefinite future. A threshold of completed-ness, for instance, was reached in Raphael's (1483–1520 CE) *Transfiguration*, so much so that it is considered by many to be his greatest work. It is therefore interesting that this supreme achievement was unfinished when Raphael died in his thirties. Geoffrey Chaucer's (1343–1400 CE) towering work *The Canterbury Tales*, likewise, is completed[2] yet unfinished. All creations become the past. If an artist walks away from a project, it becomes the past. If he dies while in the middle of a project, it likewise becomes the past. While he is working on it, more and more of his plan becomes actualized and more and more of it, thus, becomes relegated to the past: the sculptor chisels more stone, the painter adds another layer, and the composer substitutes a different arpeggio. Each step is moving a greater percentage of the project into the past, for there is less left to do.

One could say that the creator interacts with the medium to leave behind a form which will stand as an influence, aesthetic or otherwise, on the future. The hope for the creator who anticipates his death is that he will retain some of his influence *in this world* through his creative act, even though he will someday be *gone*. His life will someday become past: his tombstone will have a birth date and a date of death. The shared goal of creator and fame aspirant is thus asserted: physical death must not get in the way of continued influence.

CREATION AND THE PAST

The creator invests himself into his project and, when it is over, he steps away from it, leaving his creation behind. This is different from the lover. The lover considers past investments of the self *with respect to others* as relatively insignificant compared to his perspective on his present relationship with a beloved that is moving towards the future and full of potential. Even if he moves on to other creative endeavors, the creator, for the most part, has an interest that his creation maintain itself as the same cohesive unity it was upon immediate completion. The hope is that his creation will exist *as it was* into the indefinite future.

My own view that creators care about their objects' continuation contrasts with those who would proclaim life to be "a journey and not a destination" and those, albeit perhaps more well-read, who would agree with Dostoevsky's (1821–1881 CE) Underground Man who boldly announces that:

> Man likes to create and clear paths. . . . Perhaps the one aim of mankind is striving to achieve on earth merely lies in this incessant process of achievement. . . . He loves the process of achievement but not achievement itself.[3]

Psychoanalyst Otto Rank's (1884–1939 CE) own formidable work on creative impulses also expresses this view that the object, the achievement, is not loved or valued:

> In creation the artist tries to immortalize his mortal life. He desires to transform death into life, as it were, though actually he transforms life into death. For not only does the created work not go on living; it is, in a sense, dead both as regards the material, which renders it almost inorganic, and also spiritually and psychologically, in that it no longer has any significance for its creator, once he has produced it.[4]

The others' position is that the process (and not the object) determines creative satisfaction. These thinkers believe creators are indifferent to their creations once they are complete. I take issue with this view, although it is admittedly difficult to prove creative motivations either way.

Whereas thinkers such as Otto Rank would downplay and even discount the meaningfulness of a creators past artifacts of creation, my own view of the creator is that he, at the very least, *cannot be indifferent* to their continued existence as a unified object. And, once it is shown that indifference is impossible under most ordinary circumstances, then one may use similar arguments to draw out that he is actually *positively interested* in his creation's continuance. Of course, the creator has a new relationship with the completed work of art (because he is no longer working on it). This new relationship is perhaps analogous to our past photographs. How much life we have lived since the time our past portraits were taken seems to be a factor in whether we identify with them. Today, we may identify with pictures of ourselves at age 15 more than pictures at age 4. For some, being 15 is so distant that identification with pictures at 55 is much more likely. The connection we feel to a creation tends to be livelier in proportion to how recently we brought it into existence. Such is not the whole explanation, though.

There is another factor in addition to the contiguity of time between the creation and the creator looking backward to evaluate its significance to him. Again, we can look at picture–person identification. Whether the photograph was taken at a significant moment influences my identification with it. A picture taken at a momentous occasion, such as acting in the lead role at a high school play (age 15), is more significant to me than a picture taken eating a normal dinner at age 35. Analogously, the *Bilbao Guggenheim Museum* (which opened in 1997 CE) seems to have more significance for its architect Frank Gehry (b. 1929

CE) than his projects since. Some projects' significance to their creators are more a function of significance than of time.

It is certainly worth mention that artists keep possession of paintings (e.g. Jan Vermeer's *The Art of Painting*) personally valued as significant even when they could sell them at a high price. To make the blanket statement that the creative product has "no significance" is simply unsustainable.

When considering concepts of immortality, what average creators would think if they were deceased and observing their former world suffices to support the point: creators, on balance, would prefer that his work should persist than that their work should be destroyed. If the destruction was purposely caused by the creator, it is usually because he wants to do something better and more indicative of themselves and their talents, or that an inferior work should not take attention from the better works. For example, Michelangelo (1475–1564 CE) is said to have destroyed not less than a few images from the Sistine Chapel ceiling to make room for better ones. And, postimpressionist artists Paul Cezanne (1839–1906 CE) and Vincent Van Gogh (1853–1890 CE) frequently painted over their paintings. Pablo Picasso's (1881–1973 CE) painted over a fist and moved his horse from the center of his famous *Guernica* mural. Many of the best creators do not mind at all the scrapping of interim works to make way for better, more significant work.

One may say that this thought experiment suffices for the egoistic artist intent on "leaving something" of himself, but not for the typical anonymous artist producing on behalf of religion. If the artist does not care to sign his name to his religious work, how is it possible that he feels a personal stake in its perpetual existence? To this, I respond that those who create to perpetuate religious belief (or even those who want to safeguard their religious traditions from bad imagery[5]) would overwhelmingly prefer that their creative artifacts continue to exist well into the future. They do not seek merely to make their religion a living option for others while they are here, but they seek to make it a compelling choice for others in the future. Artifacts are testimonials. So, even the anonymous medieval artist whose Christian work was destroyed by fervent iconoclasts would be upset to learn, from his heavenly home, that his creative object perished. How heartbroken the Hindu temple builders would be to look from the beyond upon the *Qutb Minar* mosque (12th to 14th century CE) in Delhi, India, which Muslims built from the ruins of their magnificent Hindu temples.

Their artistry may have been tangibly destroyed, but their religion was symbolically destroyed. Any anonymous religious artist, from the beyond, would have *better* reason to feel worse than the egoistic artist since more than his art is destroyed and more than the reference to the self is obliterated. The belief system which was believed to transcend the artist and, in most religions, sustain the cosmos has been sacrilegiously discarded and supplanted at the same time. The threat to their faith is a threat to their ideal social and cosmic orders, which faithful creators hope will be adopted and cherished by future generations. Something much larger than any one individual is the object of attack when the religious person's contribution is nullified. The religious creator creates on behalf of his religion, to further its cause. In this way, he is like GK Chesterton's (1874–1936 CE) warrior who makes a contribution to the future state of affairs and who sometimes dies in faith that the order he helped bring about will continue. Chesterton once said, "There is no such thing as fighting on the winning side. One fights to find out which is the winning side." Even the self-consciously anonymous religious artist, creates to contribute to the winning religion, understood here as a "living"[6], influential religion.

If one believes his faith to be correct, how could he relax as others destroy that faith's influence, or worse, the faith itself? The interest in the longevity of one's faith is powerfully expressed by Emile Fackenheim responding to the Holocaust, which threatened to wipe out the Jewish religion and its people. The Holocaust, he argues, must not be allowed to wipe out Judaism:

> [Jews] are first commanded to survive as Jews lest the Jewish people perish. Second, we are commanded to remember in our very guts and bones the martyrs of the Holocaust lest their memory perish. Third, we are forbidden to deny or despair of God, however much we may have to contend with Him or with belief in Him, lest Judaism perish. Finally, we are forbidden to despair of the world as the place which is to become the kingdom of God lest we help make it a meaningless place in which God is dead or irrelevant and everything is permitted.[7]

I conclude that, in most cases, the creator desires the creation to continue. If one believes his creation is truly significant, how could he be indifferent to another wiping it out of existence? E.M. Cioran (1911–1995 CE) goes further than I do to say that one would walk away from the creative act (of writing) if he did not think his work would outlast him:

> Anyone who gives himself up to writing believes — without realizing the fact — that his work will survive the years, the ages, time itself. . . . If he felt, while he was at work on it, that it was perishable, he would leave off where he was, he could never finish. Activity and credulity are correlative terms.[8]

For Cioran, the creative activity only has meaning because of the presumed sustainability of the created product. My view, that a creator generally desires his creation's continued existence, is admittedly far short of the statement that the creator *presupposes* that creation's permanence. I do, however, argue below that the creator desires his product to exist indefinitely, without limit.

CREATIVE PRODUCTS AND LIMITLESSNESS

Creative products may indicate personal, cultural, or political strength and, as we have examined, they may be used to promote fame. When they are destroyed, the strength and influence of the people and institutions that they refer to are symbolically destroyed along with them. When they are destroyed *in form* and yet preserved *in material*, a humbling message is sent to the loser. Once upon a time, Greeks melted Persian armor for a decorative shield for a colossal Athena statue, the Bolognese transformed a regal bronze Julius II statue crafted by Michelangelo (1475–1564 CE) into a cannon, and Napoleon (1769–1821 CE) had Austrian weaponry melted to make his *Vendome Column*. The forms were destroyed, and the persistence of the material in its new form must have stung the vanquished deeply.

In the case of physical procreation, it is obvious that we desire our offspring to have continued life and influence. The procreations of our love lives, new humans, will not themselves last indefinitely. Yet the new generations of humans will, we hope, pass along human life into future time generations. Through subsequent generations' physical reproduction, we who exist now will continue at least to the degree that we contribute some genetic coding, a necessary causal link, without which future individuals of our species could not exist.

Whereas the immediate offspring of physical procreation will not live indefinitely, it is not so clear that the immediate creations of our minds will not themselves last. If one thumbs through any art history book, she will soon notice that most of the finest creations pictured within are originals, and even if they are not originals, they are not too far removed from second generation copies (e.g., the Roman copies of Greek statues). In many measurable ways, we have a better chance of directly influencing the world through mental creations left behind than we do from the descendents we leave. This becomes more and more the case the longer we are departed from the world. Our contribution to the impersonal genetic pool becomes more diluted and dubious the more generations that pass, while our potential to have our creations impact future generations remains constant (as long as the creation itself survives in unified form). It may be argued with force that the presence of the artist is more directly suggested by his work than his descendents.

This point is what Andre Malraux (1901–1976 CE) was getting at in his text *The Creative Act* when he wrote that man "longs to escape" from the "inexorable subjection" of the constant threat of death by producing works that will outsurvive the man. He asserts, "Survival is not measured by duration, and death is not assured of its victory, when challenged by a dialogue that has not yet begun."[9] The "dialogue that has not yet begun" refers to future individuals interacting with the artist through the medium of his work. Of course, if the deceased creator still has a "dialogue," he is limited in his part of the conversation by the breadth and depth of his work. His work must speak for him, on his behalf. Vincent Van Gogh had already said the same thing: "Painters—to take them only—speak to the next generations or to several succeeding generations through their work."[10] The creation left behind is able to express the undiluted voice of the artist to future generations. Of course, Malraux's remark expresses that the future people and the artist have a dialogue whereas Van Gogh posits a one way correspondence (they "speak...through their work"). Van Gogh's words are nearer to the truth, but in either case, the artist is understood as *present* in his creative legacy even as he is absent from the world of the living.

The *Symposium* arguments on love, fame and Forms endorse creativity over procreativity for yet another reason, which is that creativity comes from a different (and more refined) impulse. Diotima instructs Socrates on the matter:

> Those whose creative urge is physical tend to women, and pursue Eros by this route. The production of children gains them, as they imagine, immortality and a name and happiness for themselves, for all time. In others the impulse is mental or spiritual — people who are creative mentally much more than physically. They produce what you would expect a mind to conceive and produce. And what is that? Thought, and all other human excellence. All poets are creators of this kind, and so are those artists who are generally regarded as inventive.[11]

Of course, one might have both the creative impulse and the procreative one. Mental creativity and human reproduction are not mutually exclusive. There is, however, a point at which the two conflict, resulting in either doing neither one well or in completely forgoing one in order to pursue the other. The prolific Christian writer Soren Kierkegaard (1813–1855 CE) forwent becoming a husband and father to dedicate himself to writing. His decision was not easy and he struggled with its irrevocable consequences, but his philosophy is a widely influential one, even to agnostics and atheists. Arguably, he wrote much more and he wrote much better because of his self-imposed solitude. On the other side of denial of intimacy, history tells us of Emperor Gaozong's (628–683 CE) infatuation for his father's former concubine, Empress Wu, and how it cost the Tang dynasty emperor his reputation. Worse, it severely weakened the Chinese empire. It took his attention from statecraft to making merry. Someone who chose marriage and family and who was nevertheless a premier composer was Johann Sebastian Bach (1685–1750 CE), the   father of twenty children. Certainly Bach's music is pretty good, but had Bach chosen to foster only his mental creativity as Kierkegaard did, perhaps his music would be even better! And there might even be more of it (although that is hard to imagine). It could be argued that Bach was motivated to creative proficiency by the needs of his family. Perhaps even the early deaths of some of his children further sparked his creative output. While this may be true, and artists have certainly responded to family life with genius, my general point stands that mental creativity and physical procreativity take place in a world where tradeoffs of time and attention are constantly made.[12] To dedicate oneself to one type of creativity affects one's ability to dedicate oneself to the other, and this cannot but have an effect on creative legacy.[13]

CREATIVITY AND DEATH

The quote attributed to Michelangelo, "No thought is born in me that has not 'death' engraved upon it," reveals what even many creators fail to acknowledge. Creativity is a response to immortality's antecedent concern: death. The singer/songwriter Neil Young (b. 1945) expressed the connection also. Giving a rare interview [2005], Young detailed his walk with mortality and creativity to a *Time* magazine interviewer:

> **Neil Young:** I noticed this weird thing in my eye, like a piece of broken glass. Then I noticed that no matter what I did, it was still there. And then it started getting bigger. . . I went to my doctor, had an MRI and the next morning I went to the neurologist, Dr. Sun. . . . He says, 'the good news is, you're here, you're looking good. The bad news is, you've got an aneurysm in your brain'. . . I was supposed to go down to Nashville, so I went down there . . .
>
> **Interviewer:** You flew with an aneurysm?
>
> **Neil Young:** Dr. Sun said I'd been flying for 100 years with this thing. So I went into the studio on Thursday and recorded three songs. I wrote one on the way there and two more right away after I recorded the first one. The whole album's chronological — I wrote it and recorded in the order it appears on the record. Then I went back up to New York on Monday for a presurgery thing, flew back to Nashville, wrote and recorded songs four, five, six, seven, eight, and most of nine and ten. And then I got admitted, and they put me under. . . . There's a lot of reflection. It affected all the songs. . . .
>
> **Interviewer:** So your next album will be . . . ?
>
> **Neil Young:** I don't know. All I know is I don't want to die. I have a lot left to do.[14]

As discussed throughout this text, and particularly in the first chapter, we know we will die, and sometimes certain events bring our mortality vividly before us: the Black Death, the September 11 attacks, the death of a loved one. The death of his friend Enkidu alerts Gilgamesh. It calls his attention. Gilgamesh, *qua* man of action, responds by going on a dangerous adventure to seek earthly immortality. An aneurysm alerts Neil Young. Young, *qua* creator, adds to his creative legacy. As the *Time* journalist captions, "When the Godfather of Grunge discovered he had a potentially fatal aneurysm, he took a week, went to Nashville and added to his legacy by making another classic album." The terms 'fatal' and 'legacy' are telling. First, attention to death. Then, response to death: creativity. Renaissance artist Benvenuto Cellini (1500–1571 CE) had said it almost five hundred years earlier: "Before I die I will leave such witness to the world of what I can do as shall make a score of mortals marvel."[15] There is a race of sorts to get in everything one wants to say before the clock runs out. The creator seeks to insulate himself from total annihilation through legacy. — And, it is not sufficient to leave behind 3000 tons of Styrofoam refuse. These are footprints and signals that *a* person existed, but they are not invested with the individuality of *the individual*. Anyone can leave behind 3000 tons of refuse. Only one can leave behind a *Don Giovanni*.

Young does not want to die because he has a lot left to do. If nature acquiesced to the all-too-human plea "not now: I have a lot left to do," there would be a lot more of us living right now.[16] We all have a lot left to do because we tend to like ourselves, and therefore, we tend to give precedence to what we *could* do if granted more time. The creator Young sincerely believes that he has something important left to do and not just, say, raking some freshly fallen leaves for another season or drinking his ten thousandth cup of coffee. The creator believes he will bring about something valuable and new. He may not care if others think it is valuable and new, but nevertheless he asserts that the world will be better when he adds his valuable and new creation to it. That said, he usually hopes for some kind of acclaim, whether critical or social. I shall now examine the twin qualities that the creator strives for, the valuable and the new.

VALUE: CREATORS TRANSCENDING THE LIKELY CAUSAL CHAIN OF EVENTS

Creators try to affect their world by producing something different from what the likely causal chain of ideas and productions would have otherwise been produced were it not for the creator. The breakout from the likely path of production is what gives the creation *value*. The reason that many of the frescoes found in Pompeii are not highly regarded other than for reasons peripheral to the inherent value of the art is that the artists themselves do not manage to produce convincing images any better than other artists of the day. Worse, their pictorialism is hardly even in step with the average work created by the others. For example, there is a famous portrait of a couple from Pompeii, which although charming, is not mediocre in its execution and convincingness.

A major consideration of value, then, is that the work is beyond what might have been expected if not for the creator. Perhaps the people pictured would not have otherwise been pictured, but the execution of like-quality frescos at Pompeii could be expected. It seems that the excitement of finding an ancient city buried intact, for the most part, elevated the reputation of the works preserved in the ash, even though the aesthetic attributes of the works did not live up their acclaim.

Critics and others, (hopefully) after having enough facts, determine which creations are the most original, valuable, trend-setting, unique, epoch-making, and so on. They also find examples that they believe mark the highest achievements in a style such as 12th century *Chartres Cathedral* (High Gothic) or Raphael's 16th century *School of Athens* (High Renaissance). The creator is sometimes mindful of what the present and future critic will say, but he need not be. The creator may be doing his best, not for the ages, but for some other reason. Those who know the basic story of Elvis Presley's rise to pop culture influence will remind us that his road to stardom and creativity began when the young truck driver paid his own money to record a song for his mother. He created for his mother, not for the critic. And those who know the basic story of Franz Kafka's literary contributions will recall that his stories took form without any plan from Kafka to put what is now regarded as his best work to the public.[17]

The question of value is not just for those evaluating the significance of others' creative acts. In the mind of the creator, what makes his work worth doing is that he perceives his work to be outside of what would otherwise be done. In short, the work's perceived value is what keeps the creator interested. A young man recording a song for his mother and a grandmother making a quilt for a granddaughter each know well that their work is outside of what would otherwise be done. Their familial relation to the recipient guarantees this. It is valuable and therefore worthy of appreciation because of who did it and their relationship to the recipient.

It may not necessarily be valuable in the same way to the recipient as it might be to outsiders. One can imagine that Elvis's mother may not have fully appreciated the value in "That's Alright Mama" or that the 12-year-old girl may not appreciate the elaborate (and time-consuming) stitching patterns of her grandmother's quilting. Perhaps both recipients would focus on other aspects of value, a focus more in line with their relationship to the creator rather than the value of the creation itself. Since "my son did this" or "my grandmother did this," the recipient attaches value to the product. In other cases, due value is *not* recognized because of the relationship. If Elvis's mother listened to him practice in the family basement for six years, then this familiarity with the musician and the work might have tarnished her ability to listen to the recording with the ears of a rock critic looking for new sounds.

I leave a more complete analysis of value and relationship for another day, but I will proceed from the assumption that knowing (or not knowing) the creator may influence judgments of creations' value. The honors and acknowledgements derived from achievement are certainly tied to others' opinions, and to that extent they are beyond the control of the creator. However, the intrinsic reward that the creator bestows upon himself for a project well-done is dependent on his degree of satisfaction with how his project met or exceeded his goal of expressing value. Value is a precondition for creativity and creative legacy.

THE NEW

I reiterate that the breakout from the likely path of production is what gives the creation *value*. That the foreseeable causal chain has not been transcended in quite that way up until the time of the creation is the criterion for *newness*. It is not new if I take a bicycle seat and handle bars and make a bull's head design out of it. Pablo Picasso has done that.

In fact, it is not outside of any likely causal chain because Picasso's work puts the possibility of repeating it into the likely causal chain: into my mind and others' minds as well. So it is not new or valuable. And if I attempt to photograph his *Bull's Head* and deface it in some way to make a statement of another kind, then I am in the tradition of Marcel Duchamp (1887–1968 CE) who penciled a mustache over a print of Leonardo Da Vinci's *Mona Lisa*. I have not done any thing new.

To be sure, I *have* introduced something new if I am informed by the past, but bring about something peculiar to me, my life, or my time. For a few instances: the Italian futurist Gino Severini's (1883–1966 CE) *Armored Train in Action* plays off of the Spanish Romantic Francisco Goya's (1746–1828 CE) *Third of May 1808*. And, Goya's *Third of May 1808* seems to poke fun at the French Neoclassical Jacques Louis David's (1748–1825) *Oath of the Horatii*. The French avant-garde Edouard Manet's (1832–1883 CE) *The Execution of the Emperor Maximilian* seems to sterilize Goya's unforgettable pose, even while making the shooting occur at closer range. These four paintings, from four different periods and styles, each share formal characteristics with one another, and make visual statements about how armaments, governments, and individuals interact. Each is distinctively creative, and yet each borrows from earlier models. (Even Jacques Louis David's *Horatii,* which came first, was influenced by Roman paintings unearthed from the Pompeii excavations and Roman stories of heroic civil sacrifice.) One can be new and aware of one's traditions at the same time. There may be nothing new under the sun, but there can still be newness.

We may also see the shared formal characteristics and innovation when comparing Edouard Manet's *Olympia* to the late Renaissance master Titian's *Venus of Urbino*. Of course, Manet's central figure was rumored to be a Parisian prostitute and Titian's *Venus* a duke's wife, but a methodical copy of everything from Titian would not be creative.

In some ways judgments of newness are intertwined with judgments of value. First, there are some times when the created object is said to lack value primarily because it is not new. Most well-executed 16th century Mannerist paintings will not command the respect and price that 15th century High Renaissance paintings would because the former (quite consciously) betray their influences and, arguably, do not add much in the way of palatable newness. Secondly, what is not new is sometimes only declared so because one believes it has no value. The average preschooler's crayon drawing on construction paper is certainly new, but a value judgment influences the cruel critic of the preschooler's work to say "there is nothing new about these jagged lines and erratic coloring." In some sense, every act is new because at the moment it's being done, it is the first time in that moment that it is being done. The thing to conclude is that not everything valuable is wholly new and that not everything new is valuable. All creations deemed to be worthy incorporate newness and value to differing but significant extents. These judgments may be made by critics and relatives alike, but in his striving to be immortal, the creator's thoughts are the most telling.

THE CREATOR-PERSONALITY

The word 'art' connotes "man made." Artificial sweeteners, artifacts, and artisans all have the ability to make. The creator is concerned with the process of making (which, sometimes, includes *making destruction*). Whether obsessed or insightful, the creator's flirtations with death and immortality are worth paying attention to.

Many artists' biographies have emerged since Vasari's *Lives of the Artists*, and the accounts of certain artists' favor with popes, kings, and patrons may be contrasted with others whose introverted lives were cut off from acclaim and limelight. It is beyond doubt that the social positioning of artists had influence on their work (for example, Pope Julius II's bullying Michelangelo was a necessary cause for the Sistine Ceiling frescoes). But, as for the creative person himself and his motivations for *exercising* creativity, external influences are less important. While he may have painted due to Julius's influence, Michelangelo *painted the Sistine Ceiling masterpiece* as a result of his courageous and heroic temperament. He could have half-heartedly gone through the motions and left subpar frescoes that didn't deserve to be in the company of the richly designed Sistine walls. He didn't.

It is the creative impulse that strives at immortality. The objects left behind, though more than simply a record of consummated creative impulses, provide the narrative structure of the story of the creator's immortality-seeking. But, we must remember that Michelangelo might have created sculptures at least equal to the Sistine frescos painted during that time. His impulses happened to be directed towards painting. Khufu's (c. 2575 BCE) *Great Pyramid* could have been another, equally marvelous pyramid. He scrapped a few plans in the middle of construction before finally settling on the one that stands now. One more scrapped plan or one more round of building could have resulted in a better final product. We must not confuse the object's beauty and grandeur with the creative impulse itself. The object is there for us to see, recount, learn from, equal, surpass, respect, visit, and so on. Unfortunately, the creator's personality is not laid bare before us as are his creative products: when we examine the *Declaration of Independence*, Thomas Jefferson (1743–1826 CE) with all his individuality does not shine through. Yet, in the end, just as the products of love and fame-seeking may be traced back to immortality seeking, so may creative products be understood to follow from such a search. The immortality gained from fame, as we have seen, is dependent upon human memory. The immortality gained from creative products is dependent upon the products or, at the very least, the charitable recollection of the products.[18]

Bertrand Russell (1872–1970 CE), the long-lived and prolific mathematician and philosopher, did not hold out much hope for the resilience of human creative products or recollections of them when he wrote in 1917 that:

> All the labors of the ages, all the devotion, all the inspiration, all the noonday brightness of human genius, are destined to extinction in the vast death of the solar system, and that whole temple of Man's achievement must inevitably be buried beneath the debris of a universe in ruins.[19]

An optimist in some areas, Russell was not hopeful in the longevity of the human species or its habitat. Particularly interesting in this Russell excerpt is the brief reference to the creative impulse ("devotion" and "inspiration"). The creative impulse itself will get buried. It will be forever silenced by the individual's death and its effect is forever defused by the solar system's death. The debris of the "universe in ruins" is the same debris it would have been had the creative person never brought into being something new and valuable. The influence on the world is *as if* he had never created. Even if the debris were slightly altered by the items created in our lifetimes, this hardly resembles the immortality sought in the first place. One would never hear an immortality seeker say, "I just want to influence the final composition of the universe's junk pile." If it could be said with genuine seriousness, the 3000 ton refuse-leaver would have much to discuss with the creator.

Let me briefly take stock of the central points made about creative legacy. Creators leave a stamp of themselves in their creations, and creations are hoped to be enduring representatives of the creator long after the creator succumbs to inevitable death. The living have a significant influence as to which creations are permitted to exist, which exist in part, and which are recognized as new and valuable. Creative legacy is thus subject to the minds of the living in ways similar to fame. This explains much of the conceptual overlap suggested by the terms "famous person" and "creative person." The creator provides the object or concept to be evaluated, yet this contribution is ultimately subject to forces and trends out of the creator's control. Thus, legacy and, *a fortiori*, premeditated legacy cannot be a dependable path to immortality.

The immortality offered by creative legacy is not the immortality of continued existence. It is a lesser form, a lower bar. Yet, even so, as pointed out above, the creator cannot be assured clearance over this lower bar, since even though he contributes the creation and adds it to the world, he cannot supply the legacy. He cannot foster it. In the next two chapters, I shall explore the immortality of personality. If attainable, the personality's continued existence would seem to be the greatest possible prize to all our labors, especially if it offers an existence that is exponentially better than our lives are now. We shall now move on to the personal immortality offered through spirituality, and then, in turn, to the immortality chased by materialists and prolongevitors.

Chapter Five: Spiritual Immortality: Personal Immortality 1

Whoever eats my flesh and drinks my blood has eternal life, and I will raise him on the last day. . . . This is the bread that came down from heaven . . . Unlike your ancestors who ate and still died, whoever eats this bread will live forever. —Jesus' words from *John 6: 54, 58*

(Here is) a Parable of the Garden which the righteous are promised: in it are rivers of water incorruptible; rivers of milk of which the taste never changes; rivers of wine, a joy to those who drink; and rivers of honey pure and clear. In it there are for them all kinds of fruits; and grace from their Lord.—from the *Koran*, Surah *47:15*

Plato "immortalized" Socrates in his dialogues. Both the Socratic Method[1] and the philosopher's persona have come down to us, and history has been generally charitable to the memory of Socrates because of Plato's character development.[2] That "Socrates," the idea, is still known does not imply that Socrates, the person, still exists, or even that the idea we have of him corresponds to the person who used to exist. Anyway, do we truly seek to live merely as an idea, a concept, a memory? No. If given a choice, most of us would prefer the continued existence of our *intact personality*. We would prefer a significant continuity between who we are in this life and after death. Observing his Method and recalling his memories is a *tribute* to Socrates's person, but *not a continuation* of his person.

Yet part of what has come down to us (attached to the idea "Socrates" which we conceive when we bring him to mind) is Socrates's views on the immortality of the soul, which remain influential beyond calculation. These views speak to the confidence that Socrates had in the prospects for continued personal existence. In this chapter, I revisit Socratic and Egyptian thought, and provide an overview of the five major world religions (Judaism, Christianity, Islam, Hinduism, and Buddhism). The purpose of this chapter is to provide an overview of the influential views of the soul, highlighting the connections between our ethical duties in this life and what we might expect in the next. The spiritual afterlife is the most popular variety of immortality and, in particular, the personality's survival into the afterlife is widely believed and sought after.

SOCRATES AND PERSONAL IMMORTALITY

Some Socratic beliefs about immortality have been introduced earlier, when we looked into love and fame. To review, they are that the soul is immortal, immaterial, and capable of apprehending the Forms, which are the most abstract and primary objects of knowledge. The Forms are themselves eternal and must be so, lest knowledge be tied to the impermanent and malleable. The immortal soul, rather limitedly, expresses itself through a body. When the body dies, the soul is liberated to express itself more fully. In the *Phaedo*, Socrates is confident that the soul will exist after death. However, the Socrates of the *Apology* leaves open the fate of the soul after death.[3]

"The world, perhaps, does not see that those who rightly engage in philosophy study only dying and death."[4] So begins the *Phaedo* arguments concerning the soul's independence from the body. The philosopher, the one who loves wisdom, according to Socrates, is not concerned with the whimsicalities of the flesh, since the flesh confounds our intellectual aspirations by taking minds from the transcendent world of the Forms to this earthly world of distortion and transience. Rather, the philosopher "rightly" focuses on the immaterial Forms and values his immaterial soul far more than his material body. The soul has much difficulty comprehending the Forms, or itself, *because* of the body. Hence, the philosopher studies the separation of the soul from the body, or in a word, death. Herein lies the major difference between empiricists, who believe the senses are tools for acquiring knowledge, and the rationalist, who would tries his best to do without the bodily senses.

Even though philosophers are considered sometimes to be overly sober by laypersons (even by those that have never come across Socrates's excerpt that "the world, perhaps, does not see that those who rightly engage in philosophy, study only dying and death"), it is nevertheless important to understand why Socrates would consider the study of death to be intellectually rewarding, and perhaps surprisingly, life-affirming. The soul not only lives on after death: after death, the soul is most alive. For Socrates, death is soul's release from the body. The philosopher studies and looks forward to this moment, for this is the moment that the soul is free from the passions, impediments, and epistemic distortions that come from being intertwined with a body.[5] When the soul is freed, it is most alive given that it exists in a manner truly befitting its rational nature.

EGYPTIAN IMMORTALITY: REALISM AND LIFE IN THE HEREAFTER

The independent, vital, and potentially happy soul was taken seriously by the Egyptians thousands of years before Socrates. When one thinks of the Egyptians, one usually thinks of the pyramids. The pyramids, for the Egyptians, are not merely lasting monuments representing Egyptian architectural immortality. The pyramids are indications of Egyptian belief of a more transcendent kind: the immortality of the soul.

Egyptians had the concept of a spiritual entity, the ka, which survives death and preserves the personality. The ka is an indestructible spiritual entity, which revisits the former body at will providing that it remained intact. The ka is a soul on the move. The pyramids are monumental tombs that were built primarily to house the intact corpse, a house for the ka. Considering the swirling desert winds and the passage of over three millennia, it is somewhat of a wonder that the most famous pyramids have been preserved at least as well as the meticulously wrapped eviscerated corpses we have come to call mummies.

Within the pyramids were paintings and sculptures realistically representing the deceased. They further aided the soul in finding its body. The purpose of the pyramid, the mummified body, and the artistic realism were instruments meant to ensure survival of the ka.[6] Egyptians themselves would have considered any behavior upsetting the conditions of the pyramid, whether bandits carelessly robbing the pyramids for gold or well-intentioned anthropologists carefully exploring the burial places, a sacrilege and atrocity to the deceased. The ka had to recognize its earthly body and home. Therefore, one must not compromise the pyramid, the body, or the art. Indeed, some archeologists act on the belief that they are actually serving the purpose of the deceased's continued existence by telling their story and *keeping it alive*, but such is not the immortality the ancient Egyptian most desired. They hoped for a spiritual immortality beyond what history books and scholarly essays ever could hope to offer.

Many of the most famous pyramids are found in the Valley of the Kings at Giza, where we can find the *Great Pyramid of Khufu* (r. 2589–2566 BCE) and the alluring, enigmatic *Sphinx*. Made of a quarter million two-ton stones, the Pyramid of Khufu spans 13 acres. Of course, the Pharaoh Khufu's corpse would not need its plethora of interior space, and the grand limestone exterior would not be required to attract and sustain the ka when it returned. Yet, such extravagancies clearly were meant to reflect something of the spiritual and personal vitality that was Khufu. Khufu had power. To have the power to mobilize the estimated 100,000 laborers to implement the pharaoh's demand and master builder's plan reflects the extent Khufu's commanding influence. The pharaoh put laborers through decades of toil and mandated mid-stream building plan changes. (Of course, with Egypt over 95% desert, where could dissenting laborers go to flee from the assignment?) The grandeur of the exterior and the monumentality of the eighty pyramids, best of all reflected in the *Great Pyramid*, speak to the intensity of Egyptian belief in the perpetuity of the ka maintained within, just as the towering Cathedrals across Europe speak to the medieval fervor for Christianity.

The natural elements certainly helped maintain the *Sphinx* at Giza. For hundreds of years, the sands buried much of this lion-human monument, protecting its form from the desert winds. The head is of Khafre (r. approx. 2558–2532 BCE). At present, preservationists are implanting devises to protect the exposed likeness of Khafre from decay caused by winds. Like his father Khufu's *Great Pyramid*, the Sphinx testifies to the character of the powerful Old Kingdom pharaoh. Interestingly, recent excavations at the Bahariya Oasis indicate this hope of spiritual immortality was held by common Egyptians as well as the mighty pharaohs. A yearning to stay alive infectiously trickled down to the commoners.

The toil and building logistics of the Egyptian pyramids also conjured up immortality in the sense of fame. Figures from Herodotus (484–425 BCE) to Alexander (356–323 BCE) to Sir Isaac Newton (1643–1727 CE) to Napoleon (1769–1821 CE) marveled at the pyramids without much thought as to the preserved ka[s] protected inside. To them, as to many in our own time, the pyramids showed that monumental architecture brings fame to its patron and his civilization.[7] Moreover, with a sound building plan, the structure itself would likely prove resilient through the centuries. It is as permanent a medium as any, and as long as it remains intact, the greatness of the name remains intact. No doubt pharaohs knew that their fame would remain as intact as their pyramid. But I reiterate that fame was not the primary goal. It was welcomed, however, and it reinforced the general order of the dynastical institution. With a relatively stable society and power structure (especially compared to ancient Mesopotamia), the pharaoh preparing for his mausoleum could be confident of its preservation.

JUDAISM

The reputed founding father of Judaism is Abraham. Abraham is said to have emigrated from the Mesopotamian city of Ur to Canaan (the territory in and around the Phoenician coast) around the year 2165 BCE. The religions of the time and place in that Mesopotamian land was polytheistic (belief in many gods) and animistic (belief that spirits existed in natural objects such as streams, sun, and sand). Abraham was called by God (Yahweh) to leave that place and its religion behind for to adopt monotheism (belief in one God) and to believe that God is beyond nature (transcendent). As we shall see, Abraham is recognized as the father of all three of the preeminent monotheistic faiths: Judaism, Christianity, and Islam. Judaism maintains the following beliefs as essential: belief in a divinely inspired written word (*The Torah*), belief in a God who demands obedience to Him and justice between humans, and the belief in a homeland for the Jewish people. A narrative of the Jewish concept of immortality is somewhat difficult to craft insofar as the concept evolves with certain historical events. Even so, I shall present in outline some picture of immortality for the Jew.

No discussion of Judaism or Jewish concepts of immortality can commence without an account of the importance of a Jewish homeland. The Jewish homeland was recognized as immortal before the individual soul was. When Abraham made a covenant with God, God promised him a homeland and descendents, not personal immortality. Ethical duties were lived out for the good of the nation and the benefit of the homeland and not to earn eternal reward for the individual. Many prophets have stepped forward in the tradition to remind the Jewish people of their duties to God and each other, with the fate of their nation perpetually at stake. Moses (c. 1300 BCE) was a particularly influential and revered prophet who led the Jewish people from Egyptian bondage and frequently conversed with God. The most moving interaction between the two takes place when Moses receives God's *Ten Commandments* atop Mount Sinai and delivers them to his people, who were still wandering in the desert and quite discouraged that they had not gotten to the Promised Land of Canaan, the homeland. One can imagine the faithful receiving these divine precepts at a time when morale is low: no homeland, with trust in God and each other waning. The reconnection between God, Moses, and the people renews their faith, and they build a tabernacle, a portable dwelling place, to honor God and recommit themselves to Him.[8]

JOB AND THE SOUL'S FUTURE

The book of *Job* serves as a powerful self-image of the Jewish faithful called to trust that God knows best, even in times of sorrow, loss, and anxiety. Job, whose lifetime may have corresponded with Abraham's, indicates what kind of trust Yahweh demands of his followers. The story takes off when God and "the adversary" (the devil) argue whether Job's faith, love, and trust in God would survive the loss of blessings. As the once-fortunate Job sees his fortunes and even his family members taken away, he begins to question how it is that a man of faith, or to be clearer—*this* man of faith—could be treated with such indifference, if not divinely decreed punishment. When Job addresses God and seeks answers to his sufferings, God's response is to allude to his powers and to make it clear that Job shouldn't dare to question the ways of the all-powerful:

> Where wast thou when I laid the foundations of the earth? Declare, if thou hast understanding. Who hath laid the measures thereof, if thou knowest? Or who hath stretched the line upon it? Whereupon are the foundations thereof fastened? Or laid the cornerstone thereof; when the morning stars sang together?
> . . . Hast thou perceived the breadth of the earth? Declare if thou knowest at all.[9]

In Job's day, the immortality of the soul in the sense of a personal afterlife had not yet emerged. Abraham was not promised eternal life for his obedience to

God; he *was* promised descendants as numerous as the uncountable stars.[10] (Understandably, Abraham's being asked by God to sacrifice his son Isaac would have tested his trust in God's promise of descendents.) Without expecting a payout after earthly death, a reasonable believer would expect some assurance that God is holding up his end of the covenant. To return to Job, Job is perplexed by the *why* of his suffering. The idea that suffering can unite one to the divine (as a Christian might maintain) had not yet developed. Rather, the characters in Job (especially his three advisers) perceive his suffering as indicative that something is wrong in his relationship with God. They believe suffering is punishment for sin.

In consideration of his advisers' hypothesis, Job examines his own conscience and finds it unmarred. He is not knowingly betraying the relationship. When he asks God to explain himself (in a polite way, as a pious believer would), God does not give any details. He just rhetorically asks Job whether Job was present when the awesome world, sea, and sky were created. Thus, the story of Job provides an anticipatory allegory for the Jewish people who suffered through the pogroms and the World War II Holocaust: faithful people suffer and sometimes it seems that God is silent. This message, though, is, of course, not an answer of solace to that vexing problem of evil (*why* an all-powerful benevolent God would *permit* suffering). Faithful people suffer, so the book of *Job* instructs us, and we ought not to ask why. God's power and sovereignty over His creation qualify him to sidestep the "why" of suffering.

Although many of us hold the belief and hope that faithful people who suffer will be rewarded in heaven, *Job 42* sees Job's restoration of his fortunes in *this* life. There is no indication of eternal reward. In fact, earlier in *Job 14:12*, death is described as an intractable sleep, not a gateway to something better.[11] It is indeed important, then, for a just God to see that he sets things right in *this* life. Job lives a long life and has more children: things of this world, not of the next. Finite suffering in comparison to infinite heavenly bliss would certainly be tolerable and probably welcomed if suffering impacted one's chances for bliss ("The last shall be first"[12]). But without a conception of personal immortality, the benefit of the whole relationship is called into question when those within the faith suffer as much, and sometimes more, as those outside of it.

Later books of the Jewish Scriptures indicate the emerging concept of life in a hereafter, but, even then, some authors cannot conceive of a fullness of life commensurate with the one that many Christians and Muslims envision. For example, the forthcoming lines from *Ecclesiastes* declare that an afterlife is not assured for humans.[13]

> How can anyone be sure that a man's spirit goes upward while an animal's spirit goes down into the ground? . . . There is no way for us to know what happens after we die.[14]

Moreover, for the *Ecclesiastes* Philosopher, the land of the living is a better place than the land of the dead (except the fact that the living may observe harsh injustices[15]):

> As long as people live, their minds are full of evil and madness, and suddenly they die. But anyone who is alive in the world of the living has some hope; a live dog is better off than a dead lion. Yes, the living know they are going to die, but the dead know nothing. They have no further reward; they are completely forgotten.[16]

Tradition has it that King Solomon (r. 971–931 BCE) wrote *Ecclesiastes*. His father, King David (1007–970 BCE), is said to have written the book of *Psalms*. For his father David, there may be an afterlife, but the picture he paints is of an alternative, misty, shadowy existence replete with alienation from God. From *Psalm* 88:

> I am sated with misfortune; I am at the brink of Sheol.
> I am numbered with those who go down to the Pit;
> I am a helpless man
> abandoned among the dead,
> like bodies lying in the grave
> of whom You are mindful no more,
> and who are cut off from Your care.
> You have put me at the bottom of the Pit,
> in the darkest places, in the depths.[17]

The book of *Wisdom* similarly acknowledges a shadowy underworld (identified as Hades instead of Sheol), and it too is not a place anyone would want to visit, much less stay. But, stay we must, since "no one has been known to return from Hades":

> Short and sorrowful is our life,
> and there is no remedy when a man comes to his end,
> and no one has been known to return from Hades.
> Because we were born by mere chance,
> and hereafter we shall be as though we had never been;
> because the breath in our nostrils is smoke,
> and reason is a spark kindled by the beating of our hearts.
> When it is extinguished, the body will turn to ashes,
> and the spirit will dissolve like empty air.
> Our name will be forgotten in time,
> and no one will remember our works.[18]

One could identify the above *Wisdom* passage as existential. Existentialists are acutely aware of humans' being "born by mere chance" and of their consciously harboring the possibility of death at every moment. For the Jew, this awareness

of the brevity of life and finality of death should lead one to turn to God as creator, sustainer, and moral authority. The focus, in short, is on the eternal God and
not on the transient individual. It is remarkable that Christians and Muslims,
heirs to the Jewish traditions, will take certain precepts about the moral order,
God's love for humans, our complete dependence on Him, and use them to conceive of an afterlife worth gleefully anticipating.

CHRISTIANITY

Jesus (born approximately in the year 3 BCE) is believed by Christians to
be the Son of God. Over two billion people are Christian. Jesus was born into
the Jewish faith and a Roman-occupied land. The Promised Land, so essential to
the Jewish faith, was under the control of another. The Roman Empire of Jesus'
day had all but perfected the art of governing. Two millennia ago, when Jesus
was born, Rome enjoyed strong, centralized authority. Augustus Caesar (63
BCE–14 CE) was a strong emperor who centralized Roman government, but
was nevertheless so confident in its ultimate authority that it was often willing to
let local governors and even kings rule as long as they were effective and alle-
giant. Rome's army achieved many conquests throughout the Mediterranean
basin and beyond, which brought extraordinary wealth into the Empire's orbit.
Its impoverished and powerless masses were placated out of revolt by entertain-
ing gladiatorial contests, dependable running water, and the grandeur of Empire.
Yet the Roman way of life threatened the Jewish faith and its people: (1) Rome
stood in the way of God's Promised Land, a sovereign Israel; and (2) Rome's
continued absorption of the cultures of the known world extended Roman gov-
ernance but revealed a pluralism of cultures and faiths that threatened the idea of
a Jewish identity and even the very idea of a "chosen" people.

Rome did indeed stand in the way of God's promise to Abraham for a
homeland. There was simply stated no sovereign homeland. For the Christian,
the homeland is increasingly seen in spiritual terms. The tradition begins with
Jesus' own words, stated in somewhat cryptic terms. The Gospels recounting the
Passion of Christ (the events from the Last Supper through His crucifixion) tell
us that Jesus stated to a Roman governor, Pontius Pilate, that His "kingdom is
not of this world."[19] Does this mean that the Promised Land was a spiritual one
(a heavenly Jerusalem) all along, and not an earthly one (as the Jews had previously thought)?[20] The same book, *Isaiah*, that prophesizes a Savior's coming
still contains the prediction that God's people will resettle in their homeland *on
earth.*[21] Does Jesus take a stand on the secular matters? Is he saying that he does
not fit in with either the Romans or the Jews (who were, we may concur, also of
this world)? It is open to question and debate whether Jesus saw himself as an
agent for political upheaval in Israel.

It must be continually kept in mind, though, that Jesus was a Jew. His
credibility as the Son of God is rooted in the Jewish texts. Christianity gets its
justification from a literal interpretation of the Jewish texts that prophesize a

Messiah.[22] Without Jewish prophesy of a Messiah to come, he would at best be merely a prophet calling his people back to God. He would not be God. Jesus' profile as Son of God, however, does not entail that his words easily resolve the Promised Land question (namely, is it on earth or in heaven?). Since Rome confronted the Jewish religion and prohibited its sovereignty, Jesus would have been expected to have an opinion on whether to strive for an earthly or a heavenly Promised Land (increasingly supported by the Pharisees of the day). The fact that Jesus held many opinions, though they are not necessarily inconsistent with each other, astounded his followers and enemies alike. "Give to Caesar's what is Caesar's and give to God what is God's"[23] seems to argue for a kingdom of God *separate* from yet compatible with human kingdoms. "Thy Kingdom come, thy will be done *on earth* as it is in heaven"[24] seems to argue for a kingdom of God that should replace human kingdoms *here on earth*.

CENTRAL BELIEFS

Today, most Christians believe that Jesus is the only Son of God, will return to earth, and will judge the righteous and the wicked. This Last Judgment is the subject matter of much medieval art, including the exemplary works of the sculptor Gislebertus (c. 1100 CE) and the paintings of Giotto (1267–1337 CE) and Rogier van der Weyden (1400–1464 CE). These Last Judgments viewed God as distant, authoritative, and even somewhat wrathful, and the devil as relentlessly evil and thoughtful to make his punishments cruel. For example, Giotto shows a devil feeding on a damned soul while excreting a damned soul that he previously ate. Michelangelo's (1475–1564 CE) Sistine Chapel *Last Judgment* (1537–1541 CE), a late Renaissance contribution, illustrates the anticipated magnitude of the event. Christ, in a burst of power, decides upon the destiny of huddling, distorted humans according to their merits and demerits.

The New Testament book *2 Peter* speaks of the event's suddenness, "But the day of the Lord will come like a thief, and then the heavens will pass away with a mighty roar and the elements will be dissolved by fire, and the earth and everything done on it will be found out."[25] Jesus describes our just reckoning in the afterlife as related to how we treated other humans while we were alive. Ethics and salvation meet. To be saved, one must be ethical. What follows is the count from *Matthew's* Last Judgment scene:

> Then he will say to those at his left hand, 'depart from me, you cursed, into the eternal fire prepared for the devil and his angels...for I was hungry and you gave me no food, I was thirsty and you gave me no drink, I was a stranger and you did not welcome me, naked and you did not clothe me, sick and in prison and you did not visit me'. Then they will answer and say, 'Lord when did we see you hungry or thirsty or a stranger or naked or ill or in prison, and not minister to your needs?' He will answer them, 'Amen, I say to you, what you did not do for one of these least ones, you did not do for me.' And these will go off to eternal punishment, but the righteous to eternal life.[26]

SALVATION AND ETERNAL LIFE THROUGH CHRIST

So, salvation, in the end, is granted to the select after judgment. The idea of salvation is perhaps the single most powerful, resilient, and resonant idea to the Christian. Adam and Eve's sin separated us from God. In fact, St. Paul tells us the very existence of death came about because of sin.[27] We need someone, a human, to reconcile us with God.[28] When we are reconciled with God, sin will be forgiven and death will be conquered. God, therefore, sent his only Son to become human and to offer himself as a sacrifice for our sins. Since Jesus is perfect, he makes a perfect sacrifice. A sacrifice of something or someone imperfect would not have sufficed to bridge the chasm between humans and God. Because of the sacrifice of Jesus, even sinners like Adam and Eve may be granted continuous life in heaven with God and the saints, as seen in the Van Eycks' *Ghent Altarpiece* (c. 1432 CE), the famous 15th century oil painting showing Adam and Eve in heaven.

It is through Christ that the Christian may conquer death and gain eternal life that, unlike Sheol and Hades, worth waiting for. However, it is not fully clear to us what the Christian should expect in the afterlife beyond being in the presence of God.

How we experience the afterlife may depend on through what medium we will experience its bliss. Are we pure mind? Do we have our five senses? Do we have more? Do we have a body? St. Paul writes to the Corinthians that a spiritual body is raised from the physical one, and God chooses the resurrected body.[29] The inability of believers such as St. Paul to conceive of eternal life without some form of body leads some to lambaste those who exalt the spirit as a distinct entity only to give it bodily properties.

It is true that painters and sculptors must, in the end, represent souls as having bodies for identification's sake.[30] But this does not entail that souls *must* have bodies for them to be fully operational in the hereafter. John Hick (b. 1922 CE), a Christian, even proposes that Jesus' own resurrection may not have been a bodily one:

> In the earliest experience and understanding of the disciples, there was probably no distinction between Jesus having 'risen' and his being 'glorified', 'exalted', 'ascended to the right hand of the Father.' Less than this could hardly have launched the movement which sprang up so vigorously after Jesus' death, and more is probably not required to account for it.[31]

Certainly, if Christ can resurrect without a body, humans can too.

The foregoing shows that the Christian's hope in personal immortality does not seem to require that there really be a body to complement our soul, but it is *we* who cannot conceive of a completely immaterial afterlife. We cannot conceive of living a life beyond this physical world, but the *New Testament* contains many verses that describe heaven as spiritual rather than bodily.[32] The Catholic

Church is still very careful to shy away from descriptions of heaven that even hint at the pagans' celebrated "Cult of the body." We ought not to tarnish the imagery of a heaven with the imagery of the corrupt body. God's role is not a cosmic pleasure-maker who ensures the continuation of our bodily pleasures *ad infinitum*. As we shall see, Islam does endorse a greater connection between bodily comforts and heavenly rewards. First, Islam will (like Christianity) establish a link between ethical life on earth and reward in heaven. Secondly, the heaven of Islam (as conceived in the *Koran* and the *Hadith*) maintains, and indeed amplifies, the pleasures of earth.

ISLAM

'Salaam Alekhim' is the Muslim's standard greeting. It means "peace be upon you." The root 'slm,' standing for "peace," is hence part of the term Muslim and Islam. The connections between our duties to God, called "Allah" by Arabic speaking peoples, and duties to others are repeatedly observed by the devout Muslim. To be at peace with one's neighbors and in submission to Allah's will are inseparable. One cannot be a true Muslim without accepting one's duties to one's fellow human beings. 'Slm,' then, also connotes "submission to Allah." A Muslim is "one who submits."

When one submits to the will of Allah, Allah grants them eternal life. What eternal life is like is inconceivable, according to the prophet Muhammad. In the *Hadith*, a narration of the prophet's life and sayings, he tells his followers that Paradise is beyond conception. But, the *Koran*[33] informs the Muslim that he will get there by following the moral and theological precepts set forth therein.

MORALITY, ALLAH, AND THE PILLARS OF ISLAMIC FAITH

The view that moral duties to the human community derive from God had been endorsed by other cultures and religions. For example, Hammurabi's Code which, seeks to "make justice appear in the land" (so Hammurabi wrote), follows from acceptance of Shamash's divine command to institute justice. And, Jesus later urged his followers to see the connection between faith in religion and justice on earth when he said "Whatsoever you do to the least of my brothers, you do unto me."[34] Likewise, the five pillars of Islam oblige the devout Muslim to act on both the communal and the religious aspects of the faith. The pious believer who behaves righteously towards fellow persons is rewarded appropriately with everlasting life in Paradise.

The first pillar expresses the dominion of the one God. Muslims accept and recite the creed, "There is no God but Allah, and Muhammad is his prophet." The unicity of God had been revealed through a long line of prophets including Abraham, Moses, and Jesus. After noticing that people turned away from the revelations of the other prophets, Allah revealed himself one last time to Muhammad, considered the "seal," or "last," of the prophets. This last prophet received this message word for word, in Arabic, from the angel Gabriel. These revelations comprise the *Koran* we have today. The *Koran* is believed by Muslims to be the uncorrupted revelation of Allah, and as such, it is without peer the holiest book in Islam.

The second pillar of Islam is the *salat*, or five daily prayers refreshing the connection between the Muslim and Allah. Wherever the Muslim is, he stops what he is doing and prays. Consisting of a series of prostrations and prayers, the *salat* allows for the Muslim to be "God conscious" not only in these five segments of the day, but also in anticipation of the next prayer. The prayers are said at different times of the day according to the position of the sun, and ideally, the community of believers is unified as they pray next to each other, without benches or pews. Wherever they happen to be, whether in New York, Karachi, or Melbourne, they face in the direction of Mecca, the holy city of Islam. Again, the unity of the faithful is reinforced.

The third pillar of almsgiving (*zakat*) requires that a Muslim purify his wealth by giving away one-fortieth of his savings, or 2.5 %. Allah requires this practice in the *Koran* (so, this is not charity[35]), but the money raised has a positive impact on society and so, must not be interpreted merely as a religious exercise.[36]

Fasting (*sawm*) from sunrise to sunset during the holy month of Ramadan is the fourth pillar of Islam. This exercise, done out of love for Allah, also lets the Muslim community feel the sufferings of the hungry and should lead to more compassion (and action) for the poor, long after the month is over. Those taking part in the fast renew their sense of common purpose emphasized in each of the other pillars.

The pilgrimage (*hajj*) to Mecca is the fifth pillar of Islam. Able Muslims should make the trip to present day Saudi Arabia to circumambulate the granite, cubed Kaaba at least once in a lifetime. The Kaaba represents the connections between heaven and earth, the individual believer and Allah, and the unity of the Muslim *umma*, or community.

If the Muslim lives a life of submission to the will of Allah as stated in the *Koran*, then the Muslim enters paradise where his soul lives indefinitely without limit.

DESCRIPTIONS OF PARADISE

Like many Christians who understand the Last Judgment as a reckoning for earthly deeds, the *Koran* emphasizes that good deeds in this life lead to a satisfactory afterlife. On the Day of Resurrection, men will be judged and divided into three groups: those on the right (the blessed who will be rewarded), those on the left (the unbelievers who will be damned), and those to the fore (those brought nearest to Allah). The last group, those brought to the fore, is not discussed in detail, other than that they are near to Allah in the garden of Paradise and that their numbers will come mostly from the men of old generations.[37]

Each is presented with a book of his earthly deeds. We are told in somewhat vivid terms what happens when we receive our book. If we receive it in our right hand, then we have, on balance, lived a righteous life and will be blissful in a "lofty garden with clusters of fruit."[38] In a detailed segment, the *Koran* details some of the Paradisal perks:

> God will deliver them from the evil of that day, and make their faces shine with joy. He will reward them for their steadfastness with robes of silk and the delights of Paradise. Reclining there upon soft couches, they shall feel neither the scorching heat nor the biting cold. Trees will spread their shade around them, and fruits will hang in clusters over them. They shall be served with silver dishes, and beakers as large as goblets; silver goblets which they shall measure: and cups brim-full with ginger-flavored water from a fount called Salsabil. They shall be attended by boys graced with eternal youth, who to the beholder's eyes will seem like sprinkled pearls. When you gaze upon that scene, you will behold a kingdom blissful and glorious.[39]

The couches are described as jeweled, and the pure wine will "neither pain their heads nor take away their reason."[40] The rewarded will hear none of the idle talk and sinful speech that they have had to endure in previous life.[41]

In February 2006, Muslims around the world protested, sometimes violently, against a series of cartoons published in different European countries, including Denmark, France, and Germany. One of them showed Muhammad announcing that there were no more virgins available in heaven to be the companions of suicide bombers. Heaven ran out. The view that martyrs will be rewarded with 72 virgins, a view that some Muslims take quite seriously, is the result of patching together verses from the *Koran* and *Hadith*. *Surah 56:20's* "Theirs shall be the dark-eyed houris[42], chaste as hidden pearls: a reward for their deeds," *Surah* 56:35's "We created the houris and made them virgins, loving companions for those on the right hand," and the *Hadith's* expression that the martyr has six privileges near God, including that he "will marry seventy-two wives of the houris with dark eyes."[43] The *Koran* never mentions seventy-two virgins, and the *Hadith* does not mention explicitly that the seventy-two wives are perpetual virgins.

The Muslim adhering to the *Koran* expects heaven to be better than the greatest conceivable garden.[44] However, the eternal experience has undeniable similarities to gardens on earth. Allah instructs:

> (Here is) a Parable of the Garden which the righteous are promised: in it are rivers of water incorruptible; rivers of milk of which the taste never changes; rivers of wine, a joy to those who drink; and rivers of honey pure and clear. In it there are for them all kinds of fruits; and grace from their Lord.[45]

If one passes the Last Judgment, one enters the garden and finds that earthly relations, even marital ones, carry over to heaven (in contrast to Jesus' *Luke 20* claim that no one is married in heaven):

> And [with them will be their] spouses, raised high; for behold, We shall have brought them into being in a life renewed, having resurrected them as virgins, full of love, well matched to those who have attained righteousness.[46]

DESCRIPTIONS OF HELL

The Koranic recitation, "Woe on that day to the disbelievers" is frequently repeated in the sections on hell. We learn that hell is a place for those who neither believed in God nor attended to other humans.[47] There again is the connection, accepted by the other major religions, between true belief in God and beneficent actions towards other humans that are consistent with that belief. If we receive the book of our deeds in our left hand, then we have lived a life of disbelief and we will be chained up and punished in hellfire.[48]

First, the damned are reminded of God's power (in a fashion similar to the way Job is reminded in the book of *Job*):

> Woe on that day to the disbelievers! Did We not create you from an unworthy fluid, which We kept safe in a receptacle for an appointed time? All this We did; how excellent is Our work! Woe on that day to disbelievers! Have We not made the earth a home for the living and for the dead? Have We not placed high mountains upon it, and given you fresh water for your drink?[49]

After reciting His unmatched credentials for being in charge, Allah orders the damned to "begone to that Hell which you deny!"[50] As a permanent resident of Hell, the disbeliever is not entitled to the luscious fruit enjoyed by the blessed. Rather, his food is filth, "the filth which sinners eat."[51] He is not entitled to the shade of the tress, which the blessed enjoy. For the damned, there is no "shade or shelter from the flames."[52] Instead of greeting each other with the comforting "Peace, Peace"[53] greeting heard in heaven, the damned are unable to speak at all.[54]

The idea that our earthly lives are impermanent, but that our actions impact our eternal status after this life ends is far from foreign to the Eastern religions of Hinduism and Buddhism. These two religions focus many of their metaphysical principles on the meaningfulness of our actions and their consequences on our future life.[55]

HINDUISM

Although not as exportable as the other world religions, Hinduism continues to be the belief system of around 750 million of the world's population. It is primarily practiced by those living in India and those of Indian descent. Islam, free from the precepts of the caste system, has fared much better as far as export goes.

The Hindu caste system is more than simply an acknowledged social structure for this life. It has metaphysical justification, according to Hindus. The caste system may have been observed before the Aryan invasions of India around 2000 BCE, but it certainly became enshrined in the culture as a result of the light-skinned Aryans seeking to benefit from a system which encouraged segregation of people different from themselves. There are four primary *varna* castes, whose membership is distinguished according to ethnicity, but proponents of past and present defend the system based on the theological claim that the castes are determined by their members' spiritual development. The *brahmins* (priests), *kshatriyas* (warriors), *vaisyas* (merchants), and *sudras* (peasants) comprise the four *varna* castes. Those without a caste are called *daisyas* (outcastes). The castes, reputedly, were derived from the corresponding body part of the god Purusha from which they came:

> When they divided Purusha, how many portions did they make? What do they call his mouth, his arms? What do they call his thighs and feet? The Brahmin was his mouth, of both his arms was the Kshatriya made. His thighs became the Vaisya, from his feet the Sudra was produced.[56]

The complex theology of Hinduism cannot be easily summarized, but one outside the religion should at least understand the following: Hindus believe in immaterial, divine, and immortal souls, which every human being possesses. The soul in each of us, called the *atman*, is of the same substance as the universal soul, *Brahman*, which is responsible for our lives. Our task throughout our life (and reincarnated lives) is, basically, to get to know ourselves as divine.

> Put this salt in water, and come to me in the morning.
> The son did as he was told. The father said: "Fetch the salt."
> The son looked for it, but could not find it, because it dissolved.
> "Taste the water from the top," said the father. "How does it taste?"
> "Of salt," the son replied.
> "Taste from the bottom. How does it taste?"
> "Of salt," the son replied.
> Then the father said, "You don't perceive that the one Reality exists in your own body, my son, but it is truly there. Everything which is has its being in that subtle essence. That is Reality! That is the Soul![57]

Those who are Brahmins (priests) have the duty to be the religious leaders because they are closest to recognizing their divine nature. With such wisdom comes the social responsibility to serve as models to others. Those *kshatriyas* who are warriors, the traditional rulers and defenders of the land, have attained knowledge of their atman to a higher degree than the *vaisyas* and *sudras*. Interestingly, those *vaisyas* in the merchant group are highly regarded as the "businessmen" types of modernized capitalist societies are because merchants make a living trading the work of others. They have a ways to go in their knowledge of the religion to achieve a more worthy occupation and status. (This criticism of merchants is not as popular today as it once was as a result of India's embrace of Western capitalist principles.) The *sudras* are servants who had difficult lives, but their low standing was thought to be reflective of their actions undertaken in past lives. The caste system cannot be practically disentangled from the doctrine of the immortal soul.

Hindus do not consider the body to have importance. It is material, ephemeral, and mortal. So, one should not waste time on the worries and wants of the flesh. In an influential passage in the *Upanishads*, Prince Arjuna asks Krishna whether it is permissible for him to fight and possibly kill a family member whom he loves. Krishna instructs him that bodies dying do not amount to souls dying.[58] The material world, bodies included, is only *maya* (or, illusion): of real importance is the soul.

Birth determines caste, and each caste carries with it essential duties given expression in the *The Laws of Manu* (approx. 200 BCE). The ethical duties required of each caste, called *dharma*, are distinct from the other three. (For an important historical example, because only the *kshatriyas* could fight, the Muslims in the 11th century had a pretty easy time conquering the Indians.) When one does his ethical duty properly, he acquires good *karma*, a positive consequence for the soul. Alternatively, improper action brings about bad *karma*. Since one's life's purpose should be realizing one's divine soul and its communion with Brahman, good karma leads one closer to that goal. Through the course of many lives, Hindus are born into different castes, depending on whether the *karma* acquired in previous ones was good or bad.

In a way, the doctrine of *karma* justifies the social standing one has received. *Sudras did* something to deserve it, even if those actions that produced the bad *karma* were actions of presently unremembered past lives. The *brahmins* were, as their name suggests, closest to realizing their true nature. They had ascended to social and theological places of privilege because of what they did. So, if we return to the Arjuna warrior example, we can see that if indeed one follows his castely ethical duty *(dharma)*, then the *karma* acquired is what matters most. Supposing that Arjuna refused to fight his kinsman, he would have acquired bad karma and stained his divine soul with grime that may take many lives of diligent, caste-appropriate action to work off.

Hindus adopt a concept of immortality that combines the theological (God is in each of us), the social (we are ranked according to actions undertaken by us), and the metaphysical (beyond this physical world, there is a transcendent structure to the world and it is divinely ordered). Technically, the individual has an afterlife after each earthly life. His soul, at least, will occupy another body. The individual soul finds an afterlife at the end of all his earthly lives, but it is an afterlife in which his ego is irrevocably intermixed (and hence, lost[59]) into the divine. In the afterlife individuals are indistinct from each other. Rather, they are each part of a shared totality, which is indivisible. The question of who is married in heaven or whether we see our grandparents there has no real force since the answer is obvious. Like Arjuna, who overvalued the importance of earthly relations, those who ask about whether they will continue to be themselves in the afterlife do not really understand what it means to rejoin Brahman.

BUDDHISM

Siddhartha Gautama was born a Hindu into the rigid caste system of Nepal, India. Around 566 BCE, he was born of the *kshatriya* caste and was a son of a Sakya chief. Hindu religion dictated that the rulers and chiefs came from the warrior caste. He lived in what we would call a compound: a gated and insulated community. One day, as the story goes, Siddhartha was sitting near the gates of his compound and saw an old man, a sick person, and a corpse. The experiences of beholding humans in compromised states (death being the most compromised of all!) led him to seek truths that were unavailable as long as he clung to the artificial comforts found on his father's estate.

He then left the estate and sought enlightenment. Thirty-year-old Siddhartha decided to live as an ascetic (one who renounces material comforts to the point of self-deprivation). But, asceticism provided no enlightenment for Siddhartha, for it focused him away from the meaning of life and led him to focus on the deprivation of external things. So, Siddhartha followed the Middle Way, renouncing both the extremes of the comfortable hedonism he enjoyed on his father's estate and the austere material deprivation of his ascetic experience. Presumably, both extremes lead him to desire material comforts. An analogy might be the wealthy person obsessed with the latest gadgets modern life has to offer and the poor person fixated on his "missing" those goods: both are consumed with consumer goods even though the former alone has them.

The Middle Way suited Siddhartha well. After 49 days under a bo tree, Siddhartha found the answers he sought since the days of that awakening to suffering brought on by the sight of the old, the infirmed, and the dead men. The answers discovered by Siddhartha, now the Buddha, may be summarized in the Four Noble Truths attributed to him: 1) Life is suffering (*dukkha*), 2) Suffering has a cause, 3) The cause of suffering is craving and attachment, 4) The craving and attachment can be alleviated by following an Eightfold Path (which includes right views, right intention, right speech, right action, right livelihood, right effort, right mindfulness, and right concentration).[60]

In some key ways, Buddhism resembles the Hindu culture and faith from which it came. We are reborn until we can learn to eliminate craving and its consequence, which is suffering. When followers of the Buddha successfully identify and eliminate cravings, they attain enlightenment and become free from the cycle of rebirth. Like Buddhists, Hindus also assert the doctrine of rebirth (*samsara*) until we attain the intimate knowledge that our life in this world is not worth clinging to. Like Hindus, Buddhists assert that the external world is not worth attaching ourselves to, since it is ephemeral and pain-causing. For example, sex seems to bond us to others in a reasonably pleasant way. Sex, though, leads to children who now inherit a variety of sufferings, especially death. Moreover, sex leads us to bonds that will invariably break through the breakup of partners or by death's unwelcomed invasion into the relationship. Craving sex and marriage, then, is misguided.[61] This idea that the external world is not what it seems has a Hindu counterpart called *maya*, or illusion. Recall that the family bonds appreciated by Arjuna distracted him from the ultimate reality, Brahman.

The primary theological difference, for our purposes, is that Buddhists do not believe in the universal spirit Brahman, which we rejoin upon ending our cycle of rebirths. Other differences include the general Buddhist suspicion of hierarchy and castes within the religion. Hinduism is intertwined with the caste system. Buddhism, like early Christianity, found many followers from the lower castes precisely because it refused to respect the societal order of the time. People in low social positions were the most anxious to deny a caste structure that unduly regulated their social status, their economic opportunity, and especially their hope in a better future.

RELIGIOUS PLURALISM

Some years ago, twenty five hundred to be more precise, the Greek Herodotus (484–425 BCE) observed that different cultures treated the deceased differently. The Callatians ate them and the Greeks burned them. Of these two treatments, neither of these methods would appeal to a contemporary American who favors the embalming-then-burying treatment. However, as the late James Rachels (1941–2003 CE) argued, diverse behaviors and mores often have similar underlying values.[62] The Callatians and Greeks each tried to express their respect for the dead. They did so in their own way, but their differing cultural mores nevertheless expressed a similar underlying value: respect the dead. Could religious belief be localized modes of expressed the same divine reality? To be sure, pluralism is too often reduced to relativism: if there are too many approaches, so then there must *not* be a correct one. Or maybe, there is a "correct" one among the other competing false ones. Or just maybe, perhaps the competing religions ought to be seen as complementary expressions of the same metaphysical realities.

John Hick (b. 1922 CE) uses an argument in the spirit of Rachels's argument: diverse religions may nevertheless have the same underlying divinity. Hick argues that historical contingencies play a role in communities' attempts to understand the "infinite reality of God." The understandings are, of course, as diverse as the time-periods and communities who acknowledge them. Hick writes that the great religious traditions of:

> Moses, Zoroaster, Confucius, Gautama, Jesus, and later Mohammad, . . . the
> Hebrew prophets, the writers of the *Upanishads*, of the *Tao Te Ching*, and of

the *Gita*, Pythagoras, Socrates, Plato, Guru Nanak . . . have continued to de-
velop in larger and smaller ways through the centuries, ramifying out into the
vast and complex ideological organisms which we know as the world religions.
These religions are thus based on different human responses to, the infinite reality of God.[63]

Most of the major world religions have in common a majority of the following beliefs: (1) a belief in a system of metaphysics in which the divine order or
will is imprinted around us and within us and in holy books, (2) a belief that
immoral actions result from the misunderstanding of or the misapplication of the
divine will, (3) a belief in the extended community of humans, and (4) with the
notable exception of the early Jewish writings surveyed here, an afterlife which
reflects the deceased's successes and failings in this life (or lives, as the case
may be). In their own distinctive ways, each preeminent world religion also pro-
fesses a renunciation of this world as not being the place where we belong. The
Buddhist and the Hindu are quite firm in the view that earthly life ought to be
escaped. The Christian and the Muslim clearly favor the afterlife to this life.
The Jew, as discussed in this chapter, seems closest to feeling "at home" in this
world, but the themes of wandering, searching, and hoping are so prevalent in
their texts, that one senses in Judaism a profound alienation and palpable dis-
connect between the human heart and its earthly abode.

In the next chapter, I shall examine a conception of personal immortality
that includes the hope that we should live forever in this world. This view is
understandable from the perspective that this life is the only one we really know
and to lose it "would be," as Tolstoy's Ivan Illych said, "too terrible." Personal
immortality on earth may be sought by one without a religion of afterlife (such
as Gilgamesh), one who isn't confident that his religion will deliver an afterlife,
one who loves life and doesn't want to leave it, one who is afraid to die, or one
who is simply curious about the limits of science.

CHAPTER SIX: EARTHLY IMMORTALITY: PERSONAL IMMORTALITY 2

I intend to live forever: so far, so good.—Steven Wright

I don't want to achieve immortality through my work; I want to achieve immortality through not dying.—Woody Allen

My God, what can a man do in a mere sixty years of life? How much can he enjoy? How much can he learn? He can't even harvest the fruit from the tree he plants. He never learns what his ancestors knew. He dies before he begins to live! God in Heaven, we live so briefly!—Vitek, from Capek's *The Makropulos Secret*

Our work, even if it is creative and worthy of everlasting influence on posterity, is not us. Woody Allen, always quotable when it comes to human mortality, comedically expresses this reality. Our work is not us. It is merely a consequence of a creative life. When asked "how are *you*?" we respond (we do not answer) "busy." What we *do* for livelihoods and hobbies has come, often with our consent, to define *us*.[1] Yet what we do, even if it is creative to the highest degree, falls short of who we are and what we would most like to see continue. We ache to be more than the sum total of our work and concrete activity.

Woody Allen could have substituted 'love,' 'children,' and 'fame' for 'work' and he would have been just as funny and insightful given that none of these things are equivalent to our personality. "I don't want to become immortal through my children, I want to become immortal through not dying" is just as funny because it gets to the same point that what the aspiring immortal truly wants is his life to go on. The personality's survival into the indefinite future

79

may take two forms. One is to exist after the body dies, and another option is simply never to die. Having already considered life after death in chapter five, in this chapter, I turn attention to the pursuit of an earthly life that never ends: earthly immortality.

For earthly immortality, not just any biological existence will suffice. The personality must be intact. With the use of medical gear such as ventilators, it has become possible to keep the heart and lungs working, even after the brain has stopped working. This has brought about the term 'brain death,' which refers to the state in which a person has suffered significant, irreversible brain function loss.[2] Brain death and cardiopulmonary death can occur at different times. Debates continue on exactly how much of the brain must be dead for one to be declared brain dead, and debates even continue about whether brain dead persons have rights that other dead persons do not have.

To get to my point: one can be biologically alive and yet be brain dead, at least in the sense that one takes in air and one's blood circulates. However, we would not assume that the seeker of earthly immortality would be pleased with living in such a state, since the personality would not remain intact. For similar reasons, I will not consider one's material remains living on (e.g., one's atoms, hair, or kidneys) to constitute earthly immortality. The immortal person living on earth shall be understood as one who enjoys indefinitely continued life in which his personality remains, for the most part, linked to his life already lived and to his anticipated future life *without significant ontological transformation*.

Suppose modern medicine in tandem with healthy habits could bring about humans who could live valuable lives for an indefinite period of time and without conceivable limit. What meaning would life have? Would it be valuable to the individual living it? Would it be a good thing for society? Would it be a good thing for our species? What if, because of resource and land constraints, only some of us (but not others) could live forever? Whether societies might attain the ability to sustain an ever-growing population, in which the mean age is perpetually on the increase, includes considerations of the environmental resources, individual rights, societal fairness, and wealth distribution. Thus, questions of indefinite earthly life are of interest to philosopher, politician, environmentalist, science fiction novelist, and priest alike. They involve précising the personal benefits and harms to the individual and to society. In this chapter, I shall review the difference between limits and lifespan, and recount two fictional tales which bring to mind some of the personal, as well as social, consequences of earthly immortality.

LIMITS AND LIFESPAN

Gilgamesh, the creative product, lives, — in a way. It lives to entertain us, to instruct us about the pantheon of Mesopotamian gods. It lives to tell us about a particular Mesopotamian hero, Gilgamesh. Gilgamesh the person, even if he once existed in time and space, does not live now. If the character had his way, though, he'd be witnessing to his own experiences. He would tell us for himself how he sought counsel and help from Utnapishtim on how to live forever. He would tell for himself us about his friend Enkidu and how witnessing his friend's death alerted him to his own mortality, and how he undertook death defying adventures to meet the immortal Utnapishtim in hopes to learn how to become immortal himself. Gilgamesh would tell us that he finally obtained an immortality plant from Utnapishtim, which would have effectively extended his lifespan indefinitely, but that he lost it to a serpent. Of course, he would never be able to tell us this last part of the story since he lost the plant to the serpent. Because of this loss, he was stuck with the human lifespan.

Humans' average lifespan is about 100 years[3], with its maximum lifespan about 122 years[4]. Of course, as a group, more and more of us are approaching the human lifespan's upper limits. In statistical terms, an individual randomly chosen out of humans born in 2000 has a greater probability to live longer than an individual born in 1970, who in turn, has a greater probability to live longer than an individual born in 1940. Barring pandemic disease or other catastrophe, there is a correlation between public health, private habits, and life expectancy. As our public health endeavors succeed and our private habits improve, our "life expectancy" *as an aggregate group* tends to increase. We cannot, however, expect an individual life expectancy to go beyond the limits of longevity that the human lifespan affords us. Lifespan is in domain of the possible and life expectancy is in the domain of the probable within the confines of the possible.

Picture a healthy NBA champion basketball team asked to play at full effort against a talented, NCAA Division II team. The NCAA team might reasonably expect to "stay in the game" for two minutes. On an extraordinary day when the NCAA team comes in at top conditioning, they may be able to compete for longer. However, we would never expect the NCAA team to win against the superior NBA team or force the game to continue into indefinite overtimes. Analogously, we cannot beat death nor live on "borrowed time" indefinitely.

But what about Biblical figures who are said to have lived up to an incredible 969 years? It is true that some of the numbers seem so inflated that we can scarcely imagine their truth. Differing speculations abound about how the numbers came to be so extraordinary, with one possible explanation being that the writers of these stories measured years differently. Alternatively, perhaps the writers in later eras asserted the greatness and worthiness of their ancestry in the currency of years lived (and hence, to emphasize their own worth-by-pedigree). Thus, extended time on earth indicates power over nature, favor with God, and overall extraordinariness compared to other humans. Or, the embellishment of dates may be trying to tell us symbolic truths rather than historical truths.

One Biblical character has come to stand for indefinite earthly life. Methuselah, the oldest man on record, lived for 969 years.[5] His own father Enoch, though, never died (he was literally "transformed," and "taken away.").[6] Methuselah's life is said to have coincided with the Expulsion from the Garden of

Eden, and his grandson Noah's saving Arc. One might even say he looks pretty vibrant in the *Canterbury Cathedral* stained glass panel: he was, after all 187 when he had his first child, and he lived 782 years after that![7]

Whereas medical researchers work to cure diseases such as heart disease, cancer, and AIDS, increasing life expectancy within the confines of lifespan, Methuselah's name has come to be associated with challenges to the human lifespan itself. If major diseases were eradicated, the benefiting humans could expect to see increases to their average life expectancy. If Methuselah projects were successful, the benefiting humans could be heirs to a longevity far exceeding the limits of the current human lifespan.

Although the time period in which Methuselah lived was most likely a difficult one (with reckless sinning and catastrophic flooding), his name conjures up optimism and nostalgia for a return to a golden age of sorts, a golden age that never really existed. For example, Science fiction writer Robert A. Heinlein (1907–1988 CE) tells of "Methuselah's Children," born of many generations of unions of persons with good genes for longevity.[8] And, playwright George Bernard Shaw (1856–1950 CE) chose to name one of his plays *Back to Methuselah*, but like the scientists working on extending lifespan, Shaw looks to future ages to bring about the return to happiness and long life. Yet, the 20th century golden age sentiment associated with Methuselah's time has waned a bit in its more contemporary 21st century uses, given that theorists are aware of potential problems that would be the result of too many Methuselahs. "Back to Methuselah" had been optimistic, but recent theorists sound the more alarmist more alarmist sentiment "Coping with Methuselah."[9]

PROLONGEVITY PLUS FOR THE INDIVIDUAL:
THE FEELING OF IMMORTALITY AND THE MEANING OF LIFE

George Bernard Shaw's Methuselahs live into their 300s. I am aware that 300s, or 960s for that matter, is not equivalent to not-dying (objectively speaking). Someone who dies at 333 has a birthday and a death day, and is not, strictly speaking, biologically immortal. But, individuals with this "prolongevity plus," this indefinitely long life without clear limit, would tend to feel as immortal as any teenager would. Youth, understood as a feeling that the individual has a significant time period to live until death, is usually on the side of a 200 year old, when one will live a few hundred more years. He who lives with access to death-postponing remedies is no less convinced of his limitless, indefinite future than the fame-seeker is convinced that he will be remembered once he achieves fame. So, remember that a person would have to be immortal himself to appreciate his true, objective immortality. I am not, in this book, directly assessing our prospects for true immortality.[10] Rather, I am examining ways of thinking about immortality and assessing our concepts of it, keeping in mind the introductory point that no one has had direct experience of objective immortality.

The feeling of earthly immortality may be dreadful, fantastic, or anything in between, depending upon one's feeling about the meaning of life. If life is meaningless, the extension of it could be dreadful. If life is packed with meaning, the extension of it could be fantastic. What gives life its meaning?—Not any life in the general, abstract sense, but *your* life and *my* life.

We could justify our existence by pointing to the service we give to others and to our civilization. On the other hand, if living for others were the *primary* and *eminent* determinants of meaning, then our individual lives could very well lose their meanings (and possibly, our claims to civil protections) when we cannot offer service to others and, instead, become a net drain on them. At the very least, an answer that defines the self's meaning in terms of something outside the self minimizes the self in the manner of Neo-Darwinists who observe the individual's purpose merely through its service to species.[11] Life becomes about projecting genes into the future, but the question "why life at all?" gets discarded before it's considered. It is indeed worthy to wonder why we, even as part of a greater whole, ought to extend individual life to future individuals if individual life has no inherent meaning.

We could justify our existence by pointing to the next life. This earthly existence has meaning because of the next one. We are on trial in earthly life: sufferings, accomplishments, good deeds, devilish ones, thoughts, and cares test our worthiness for the fruits of the next life. But here, like the evolutionary theorist who justifies the self in terms of another, we perpetuate confusion and obfuscation. How does the next life supply the answer sought, "Why life?" As Wittgenstein wonderfully puts it:

> Not only is there no guarantee of the temporal immortality of the human soul, that is to say of its eternal survival after death; but, in any case, this assumption completely fails to accomplish the purpose for which it has always been intended. Or is some riddle solved by my surviving for ever? Is not this eternal life itself as much of a riddle as our present life? The solution of the riddle of life in space and time lies outside space and time.[12]

Many contemplative individuals seek meaning without reference to beings, systems, or processes outside the self. Many never find it. (And, some who think they've found their meaning should probably have kept looking.) Perhaps it is premature and presumptuous to assume that an individual can find the meaning for one's own life: that which makes *one's own* life worth leading, but we may nevertheless examine a few considerations.

Two traditional answers have been given for why one's own life should have meaning. The first answer is that earthly life, like any thing else that is impermanent, has some meaning because it does not last. The second answer is that only things that are permanent have meaning, since they are stable and able to be counted on. Thus, earthly life is not meaningful, or at the very least, it is not as meaningful as it could be if it were permanent.

THE FIRST ANSWER: IMPERMANENCE AND MEANING

The 20th century existentialists celebrated the mystery of the fleeting. Our spark of human existence, of our being a being-in-the-world, flickers with an eternity of nothingness both before us and after us. Existentialists believe that we ought to make our individual existence special and give it meaning through choice and creations that reflect who we want ourselves to be: we ought to make the real conform to our ideals. Many tended to de-emphasize God as the architect of the ideal. As Jean-Paul Sartre (1905–1980 CE) explains, in *Existentialism is a Humanism*, there is very often a certain ambiguity in religious commands that leaves the practical application of biblical injunctions to the agent carrying them out. So, even one who acts in religious modes must bear the total responsibility since it is the individual, and not God, who chooses to follow religious precepts. The agent, then, is responsible for asserting himself in the world and for translating any ideals he has from his mind into his behavior. We have but a brief opportunity to write the record of our lives. We ought not to let others do it for us, and we become the judges who evaluate whether our concrete actions correspond to our ideals.[13] The Last Judgment scenarios of Christianity and Islam, with God separating the worthy from the wicked in imaginative ways according to His ideals, become internalized, only in the internalized scenarios, human beings create their own ideals judge themselves according to them. Being mortal, we have a limited time in which to act and we must make good use of our time. What is difficult (or even impossible) to hold onto is seen as precious in this analysis, precisely because we have a limited time to define ourselves. One may think of a senior prom, college athletics, a first love, and so on.[14] Usually someone who has already gone through these events stresses the events' significance as another, perhaps a son or daughter, partakes in their own fleeting activities.

THE SECOND ANSWER: PERMANENCE AND MEANING

Others argue that life has meaning because it is permanent, even if the soul now exists in this fleeting world. Followers of Pythagoras, Socrates, and Plato endorse turning attentions away from this world to find meaning beyond it. The person must die to free his soul. Most major religions, including Christianity, Islam, Hinduism, and Buddhism, support the notion that the permanent spiritual identity of humans matters far more than the transient biological identity. We have souls and our souls have the potential for everlasting life. The body does not have such everlasting life, and acts done (including the act of "having faith") while the soul is in the body do impact the kind of everlasting life to which we have access. When Jesus said, "For whoever will save his life shall lose it; but whosoever will lose his life for my sake shall save it,"[15] he wanted his followers to know that preserving the spiritual life comes at the cost of giving up the earthly one. The abbot St. Benedict (c. 480–c. 547 CE) considers the tradeoff a good deal. The eternality of the soul led him to argue, in his *Rule* for monks, that we should confidently trade off this life of the world in exchange for continued spiritual life in the next:

> And if we want to attain eternal life, escaping the penalties of hell, then while there is yet time, while we are still in the flesh and able to fulfill all these things before darkness and death come upon us, let us hasten to do now what will benefit us in eternity.[16]

Blaise Pascal (1623–1662 CE) later proposed his famous Wager argument which also urged Christians (and others) to consider this life that Gilgamesh so craved as expendable in comparison to the infinite one in heaven:

> Let us weight the gain and the loss in wagering that God is. Let us assume these two chances. If you gain, you gain all; if you lose, you lose nothing. Wager, then, that He is. . . . There is here an infinity of an infinitely happy life to gain [and] a chance to gain against a finite number of chances to lose.[17]

A life of (Christian) faith implies the primacy of the infinite. This view extends to other faiths, such as Islam. Some, upon learning that the Jordanian born Al Qaeda leader Al-Zarqawi (1966–2006 CE) was killed in May 2006, said things like, "Now he is a martyr; praise God." If you live for the faith (for a finite period of time), then you are an heir to Paradise. Any gambler would take those odds (and, as we know, gamblers are at best only semi-rational!). The exchange of bodily, finite well-being for the spiritual, infinite well-being is a compelling proposal, which cannot be falsified since no one has come back from the dead to say, "my sacrifice of the finite wasn't worth it: there's no life after death!" The man of faith usually will not go so far as to deny that this present life has any meaning whatsoever, but when compared to an eternity with God, his finite self is no match. Who would spend his temporary life in the flesh doing things that might make his spirit fuel for the raging fires of hell when he could spend it doing things that would earn his soul eternal bliss in the presence of the Blessed?

The religious person thus understands the meaning of earthly life in terms of spiritual life. Indeed, without these terms of spirituality, many religious persons are at a complete loss to explain why we are here. The Platonic philosophical tradition, as we have seen, also eschews the world. Most people understand questions about the meaning of life to refer to the earthly one: why are we here (on earth) in this biological life of ours? People who understand the meaning of the term 'life' to be biological or spiritual usually answer that the meaning of life is to be found within the transitory or permanent, respectively. The spiritually minded person, however, is nevertheless interested in issues of life on earth even if he finds ultimate comfort in the beyond. How he behaves on earth may impact his chances of infinite reward.

For example, many bystanders, citizens, and politicians who stood behind the Schindler family to continue Terri Schiavo's (1963–2005 CE) tube feedings came from religious perspectives, which view actions taken *in this life* to be, at the very least, relevant indicators of true belief. Schiavo, recall from the 2005 publicity, was the young woman declared brain dead by many doctors, given many years of rehabilitation opportunities, and who had arguably, in conversation, declared in her lucid days that her will was to die if she ever existed in such a vegetative state. After years of court battles, her husband received legal permission as her guardian to withhold the feedings necessary for Schiavo's biological survival. Indeed, no one has argued that Terri Schiavo's life was destined for earthly immortality had she continued to receive nourishment. But, again, actions others took with respect to Schiavo impact on their own prospects for the next. Ironically then, the wrangling over Schiavo's continued life had much more to do with what kind of continued life her husband, her parents, and the religiously motivated people wanted for themselves. All the same issues impacting the earthly immortality debate were expressly present in the Schiavo case: life quality, life extension, social resources, individual autonomy, family influence, and state intervention. Please note how these same issues that affected perceptions in the Schiavo case will be central to the cases of prolongevity which I discuss next.

PROLONGEVITY WITH AGING: THE CASE OF TITHONUS (CASE 1)

Aurora loved Tithonus, but there was a slight problem. She was an immortal goddess, and he was a mortal human. So, the goddess asked Jupiter to make her lover Tithonus immortal. Jupiter agreed. However, Aurora forgot to ask Jupiter that Tithonus stop aging. Tithonus, therefore, gets what might be considered a horrific gift: he ages eternally, yet never dies. Playwright James Merrill (1926–1995 CE) imagines Aurora's delivery of this mixed news to Tithonus, just after the newly minted immortal Tithonus chides his father for being mortal:

> **Tithonus**: Oh Father, even if you live another ten, another twenty years, even if you were my age — you'll dry up and die, each year older and sicker, and your mind gone! And I'll be as I am now, strong, young, a hundred years, a thousand, after you're in your grave! . . .

> **Aurora (To Tithonus):** Darling, I'm frightened. You said something just now...Darling, there's nothing in it about not growing old!

> **Tithonus (not understanding):** What?

> **Aurora:** Perhaps it doesn't matter. I hope it doesn't matter, but — you know, you won't stay young. You'll never die, but — well, you'll grow old, naturally, the way people *do*. . . .

> **Tithonus (*aghast*):** But that's the whole point!

> **Aurora:** You didn't ask for that! You never said you wanted to stay young!

Tithonus: Then you've *never* understood!

Aurora: *You* never bothered to explain!

Tithonus: I knew it was too simple! I said so, didn't I? But you smiled and — You can have it changed, you can ask again!

Aurora: No . . . I'm afraid not. . . .

Tithonus: But you must!

Aurora: I can't. Once only . . .

Tithonus: But what will become of *me*?

Aurora: Oh my dearest, my love — what can I say? That's my fault — does that help? It's a terrible thing, I suppose, but it doesn't change us! I don't see that it does! I'm yours, entirely, eternally....

Tithonus: Don't say that! Think what I'll be in — Oh God, less than a hundred years! A horrible old man, drooling, deaf![18]

Tithonus goes from thinking how "strong" and "young" he will be a hundred years after his father is dead to how "old, drooling, and deaf" he will be in a hundred years. Tithonus lives the worst of infinities as he forever approaches death without arriving at it. He is like Zeno's (c. 5th century BCE) Achilles who forever approaches the finish line, but never finishes the race. As expected, Aurora soon loses romantic interest in Tithonus, but allows him to stay alone at her empty palace while she is gone. The poet Alfred Tennyson (1809–1892 CE) expresses how Tithonus, unhappy being a house pet, must have pleaded to the gods for death. Tithonus begs:

Release me, and restore me to the ground;
Thou seest all things, thou wilt see my grave[19]

The Baroque painter Francesco Solimena's (1657–1747 CE) rendering of Tithonus shows the unhappy immortal shielding his eyes from the light of Aurora and her crown. (Perhaps had he been younger, the light would not have bothered him so much!) Indeed, aging can be difficult: we shrink, our metabolism slows down considerably, our skin and hair lose volume and luster, our lungs and kidneys have compromised functioning, our reproductive capabilities weaken or cease altogether, our vision and hearing and taste are much less sharp, our immunity is not what it used to be, and our mind operates with depleted brain cells.[20] If we kept losing faculties forever, it would give new meaning to Bob Dylan's lyric "Just when you think you've lost about everything, you find there's something else to lose."

It is pretty clear that Methuselian enthusiasts would prefer to *arrest* aging and extend life rather than to *continue* aging and extend life. If they could not arrest aging, then it would only be a matter of time before the recognizable personality would be gone and we wouldn't have the immortality sought. The resultant living agent would not, therefore, be equivalent to the previous one, given enough time. James Merrill's Tithonus, as we have seen, wonders "What will become of *me*?" He does not think he will be extinguished in all possible senses, but in his question he acknowledges that the survival of his *personality* is in jeopardy. In Shaw's play, *Tragedy of an Elderly Gentleman* from his *Back to Methuselah*, the people a century or two older than the elderly gentleman have much more spring in their steps. Unlike Shaw's technically-younger gentleman, they do not have to rest so much, and they do not get confused so easily. They retain what is most essential: they retain their personalities. Tithonus, however, is not so lucky.

With aging comes the decline of mental faculties, and additional social and moral considerations arise from prolonging lives indefinitely. There are two modes of thinking which inform our moral considerations on how we will approach and decide the value of prolongevity and personhood. We are heirs of Enlightenment thinking, which considers personhood coextensive with dignity and Reason. But, we also inherit the religiously inspired, but no less American, notion that personhood is a gift from God, which humans must respect: "We are endowed by our creator with certain inalienable rights..." On that view, reason does not seem necessary for personhood. Is Reason primary?, or is God's will primary? How do we know? Some Reason celebrants would argue that the individual who mentally declined below a certain low threshold is no longer a person who deserves the fullest moral consideration. But then what of infants? What of people sleeping? Or drunk? Surely their mental lives are compromised. Is it the irreversibility of the incompetence?

While some of these questions eventually may be sorted out to satisfaction, even more difficult concerns await those who put God's plan and the Ensoulment (i.e., the giving of a soul to each person) of humans above Reason to support prolongevity efforts. The soul in embryonic stem cells, the soul in the youthful body, and the soul in the demented, Alzheimer's patient each possess infinite worth in the eyes of God. If Reason and personhood are disconnected, then the Ensoulment celebrants would have to accept life extension, and even perhaps do all they can, within the moral precepts of "help the less fortunate," to extend all permutations of human life from blastocyst through brain death. This certainly gives them less leeway to make judgments about weighting resources towards those with a greater mental prognosis and away from those whose mind and "quality" of life is not likely to recover.

PLANNING FOR AGING AND PROLONGEVITY

Skin care products may make one "look" younger, but they will not make one "be" younger. Medicine may prolong one's life and even give one "new parts," but the Thesian ship of the body, considered as a whole, ages.[21] As of this book's writing, there is no way to prolong life while at the same time arresting aging. Our society continues to inch closer to a Tithonusian state of affairs, with an aging population having more and more options to prolong biological life. John Hardwig, a philosopher from the University of Tennessee, wrote an essay defending the seldom-defended claim that the old and ill may sometimes have a duty to die. Duties, as we have learned from our Kantian heritage[22], are binding whether we want to do them or not. The aged may not want to die. They may feel they have a lot left to do. Some cultures, usually non-Western ones, may reinforce their feeling that their existence is valuable even if it is a net drain on social resources. For example, the Japanese families lucky enough to have a great-grandfather around will not waste opportunities to honor his presence. As science and medicine bring about increased life expectancy, we need an ethics that is capable of being at once sensitive to the individual, society, species, and environment. Harding attempts to begin a formulation.

Tithonus wanted to die. He could not find value in his continuous, incremental aging without death. But suppose he didn't want to die. Suppose he liked sitting alone at Aurora's palace and living off the kindness of others. Saying that "there is a deep irony in the fact that the very successes of our life-prolonging medicines help to create a widespread duty to die," Professor Hardwig asks would-be prolongevitors to deliberate about, among other things, the following, which I supplement with considerations relevant to Tithonus:

1) Whether continued life would be a continuing emotional or caregiving burden.
Tithonus is said to have lost the use of his limbs and could not, then, gather his own food. Yet, he lived off food fit for the gods. He may have been relatively easy to look after, not because his health afforded him independence, but because of Aurora's status as a goddess. She could do more for him than others could. However, most middle class families would not leave an immobile loved one alone all day the way Aurora did, nor would the members of the middle class have the means to provide the best possible nourishment without significant additional sacrifice. A modern day Tithonus would cause hardships to many ordinary families. Financial burden soon would trickle to the established social network.

2) Whether he already lived a full, rich life.
Tithonus came from a regal Trojan family. He was the son of a king, Laomedon of Troy and also the father of a successful son, Memnon, who went on to become a king of Ethiopia. Tithonus was beloved of a goddess and had a share in

goods unattainable by most mortals: courtly life, money, power, influence, good company, and so on. This certainly qualifies him as having lived a full, rich life. Hardwig would say that an aged Tithonus, if he could die, is more likely to have a duty to die, since he has enjoyed so many goods already.

3) Whether loved ones have already made significant contributions to him.
The past kindness shown to Tithonus in terms of shelter and food entail that there is significant contributions to him have been made. This means that further favors, perhaps, ought not to be sought. How this consideration applies to real life is difficult to say. Does the 74-year-old diabetic cared for by his wife for the past 20 years have more of a duty to die? Wouldn't the person's death in some way devalue the sacrifices made over the past 20 years? What about the wife's emotional investment? How should we honor the values of spousal emotional connectedness, past investments, the fulfillment of the marriage vow to the "edge of doom" (to use Shakespeare's words)?

4) Whether he could improve his situation so as not to require so much aid from others.
Like many terminal patients, especially those with degenerative diseases, Tithonus cannot conceivably do much more to improve his situation and reassert the independence he once had in his younger days. His future would include more inevitable aging and, therefore, any strides made would be cancelled out eventually. Of course, the aging persons could make changes to their diets, habits, and attitudes, which could decrease the amount of external support needed. If they did succeed in improving their situations, then this lessens the probability that a duty to die is present.

5) Whether he could continue to make positive contributions to the others.
The aging can offer advice, kind words, experience and a sense of history and positively impact the lives of others. This must not be underestimated, even in our own culture which tends to be drunk on youth. If Tithonus, or any mortal considering indefinite prolongevity, can overcome curmudgeonism and actually enhance the lives of those around, then this lessens the probability that he has a duty to die.

6) Whether his personality, that made him loved, is still reasonably well intact.
With the inevitable decay of the mind that accompanies the body's decay, the aged person may not be identical to his previous self. This question of identity requires complex philosophical analysis beyond the present book's scope, but a person's loss of memories, dispositions, and character traits, might disassociate him from his past which would then "take away the person's agency and the emotions that bind [him] to others."[23] If one knew that such a loss of agency

would come in a relatively short time, then he may have a duty to die, according to Hardwig.

7) Whether his actions in the past were wasteful and contributed to his current reliance upon others.
In Tithonus's case, he did not fail to ask Jupiter for everlasting youth. Aurora made the mistake of not asking for both at the same time (which, the Tithonus of James Merrill said, was "the whole point"). Had the failure been his, Tithonus would have had less of a claim to enlist aid from others. If a person spends money without saving for old age or illness, that person would have less of a claim on aid from others. Past actions sometimes put us in our present situations and the consequences of our negligence must be faced.

PROLONGEVITY WITHOUT AGING: THE CASE OF ELINA MAKROPULOS (CASE 2)

The continual upkeep of mental faculties in the face of aging is, at the moment, unlikely. The body breaks down without discrimination. If brain and body are as connected, as materialists believe, then it might be practically impossible to maintain sharp mental faculties amidst the same forces that break down the bodily machine. If it were possible to keep the mind sharp but not the body spry, many still would not want to live an infirmed life that would preclude enjoying the simple things previously enjoyed: for example, nature, sport, conversation, or listening. But let's say that we could live longer without experiencing the infelicities commonly associated with aging. Social and moral concerns would still remain. Where would we stop the aging, if we could? We could stop it at the biological equivalent of eight years old and perhaps solve any impending overpopulation crisis resulting from an ever increasing society of reproducing immortals. But given the volume of love poems and love paintings, and concluding that there is a glory to love and parenthood, we may not want to deny future generations these experiences. If we stop aging at twenty one, we might have to implement a cap on the number of children couples are permitted to have, and we might have to set the limits quite low given the likelihood that the offspring from the couples will themselves live indefinitely and reproduce other immortals.[24]

Karel Capek, a 20th century Czechoslovakian playwright, considers many of the individual and social consequences of such prolongevity in his *The Makropulos Case*. To summarize the story, a beautiful opera singer has been alive for 337 years, but appears to be only thirty four. Her voice is perfect, her looks attract gazes, and her knowledge (especially historical knowledge) is close to perfect. How can this be? Her father had developed an immortality elixir while serving as court physician for Emperor Rudolf II, but the emperor wanted it tried on the physician's own daughter first to make sure it wouldn't kill him when he took it. And so it was that Elina Makropulos from Crete begins her immortal life that would span over three centuries and various personas (she changed her name and identity more than a couple of times saying, "One cannot live among you people for 300 years with the same name"[25]).

The social consequences of one Makropulos would not seem to be overwhelmingly negative. In the play, we even learn of a few others that took the elixir, and their existences do not seem to create social upheaval. Of course, one opera singer, much younger (in actual years) than Makropulos, thinks of quitting the profession because she'll never compare to Makropulos. That is surely a pity for the aspiring singer, but this sort of envy and hard feelings are ever-present even without immortals among us. One could be jealous of the talented (and rich) actor who retains his dashing appearance in spite of the decades, and one can be spiteful of the gifted singer who through natural talent, graceful looks, and a bit of luck, carries himself as if success were a birthright. At the end of Capek's play, when others learn of the elixir and begin to wonder whether they should hoard it for themselves, or share it with mankind, or destroy it altogether, the social consequences of scores of immortals becomes highly salient. Who would agree to marry for 300 years? And, of those, who would fulfill the agreement, especially given today's high divorce rates? Should we limit the availability of the elixir to those who can afford it? Or, to those who will make the most of it? Capek's Prus here enters his elitist vote on this question:

> Please, I do not want to argue. But, if I may: the ordinary, small, stupid human being never dies. A small person is everlasting, even without your help [of the immortality elixir]. Smallness multiplies like the rest, like flies or mice. Only greatness dies. Only strength and talent die, because they cannot be replaced. It may be in our grasp to keep that alive. We can begin an aristocracy of the everlasting.[26]

The thought that the most excellent should be the most eligible for everlasting life can lead to or follow from racism, to which Charles Lindbergh (yes, the pilot) and Dr. Alexis Carrel (the Nobel Prize winner) seem to have subscribed. The two thought earthly immortality possible by replacing broken organs like engine parts.[27] Makropulos herself, social considerations aside, is unimpressed with her life, even though her talent and renown impresses all the others. She seems unmoved by the attention given to her talent, personality, and beauty as evidenced by her frequent yawning and boredom. She does not even take joy in erotic companionship. Makropulos, in these ways, may be seen as an example that life has meaning because it is impermanent: when life is permanent, life is meaningless[28]:

> **Makropulos:** For you, everything has meaning. For you, everything has value because for the few years that you are here, you don't have time to live enough. God, if I could only once more . . . (*She wrings her hands.*) Idiots! You are so happy! You disgust me with your incessant happiness. And all because of this silly chance, that you are going to die soon![29]

Although, on the contrary, it may be that Makropulos was unable to keep herself interested in enough new things and this was the cause of her unhappiness. On this view, it was her inability to cope with her immortality and not extended life *per se* which was to blame for her intolerable boredom. With all the things of this world to discover, to know, to solve, to love, it is difficult to believe that Makropulos could only find joy in the first century of her life.

In the late 18th century, Englishman Thomas Malthus (1766–1834 CE) predicted that the world's resources could not sustain the predicted population much beyond 50 years from when he wrote. He was wrong. Sometimes predictions of gloom do not materialize. Even with this lesson of history in mind, it is intuitively obvious and research-supported that population age structures and increases do play roles in economic development.[30] And, economic development influences healthcare, education, and standards of living. Capek fits considerations of resources into his play. Near the end, Vanek hypothesizes that we may have to abruptly end some immortals' lives just to make space for others' enjoyment of worldly goods. If life continued without limit with reproductive faculties and freedoms intact, our population growth and, consequently, peoples' access to real estate and a host of other goods would lessen as time went on. This sets up quite a different dilemma from triaging resources towards those with the greatest life expectancy. In this scenario, other factors besides potential years to live would be the difference-making factors. Now, the potential life to be lived for one immortal is the same as for another.

Perhaps we can establish a method of triage not on how much time is predicted to be ahead of the agent, but on how much time has been lived. Children, for instance, can usually be talked into relinquishing a toy when we speak in terms of having had the toy for a long time. They should, therefore, "give someone else a turn." But children, as we know, may, on any given day, be inclined to say "I had it first" and listen to no other reasoning that asks them to override this fact.

Life is not like toys. Life is the precondition for having any goods whatsoever. Most people would not give up their lives (everybody "has their own life first") even if they would give up their toys. And, it is not clear that they'd give up their toys. Toys are something a living being uses. Yachts, stocks, land, cars, food, and clothes are not given up easily simply on the basis that the owners have had them long enough. There are many people in this world of ours who have never refrigerated their food, driven a car, or woke up in a beach house. Do these "deprived" persons have a claim against those who continue to enjoy these things simply because the latter have had them long enough? Would we really think that immortal citizens would lay down their lives for the good of the collectivity? The well-to-do, which includes most readers of this book, could plead the "I've worked for it" response to giving up our toys. It is therefore a right to continue to enjoy them until their voluntary parting. So, would politicians or courts decide based on numbers and trends when to require a death of someone who has had life long enough? Notice that "to live" and "to have life" are different ways of saying the same thing, but the latter implies that life is a forfeitable possession.

Of course, no one could plead the "I've worked for it" when asked by outsiders to give up our lives on behalf of some abstract principle of fairness between living beings. Birth will always remain a non-choice for those born. We don't work for birth (if we did we would have to preexist ourselves). Yes, there is nothing that we do to earn existence. Only if the earthly immortality enjoyed was achieved merely by those who worked to maintain a health and fitness level threshold could a person invoke a right to life based on personal merit. In the case of an immortality elixir, the Capek kind, there would not be such a requirement of health and fitness. In the case of an elixir paid for as a product in a privatized health care system, a person could link his right to continued life to the fruits of his work. "My education got me this job, this insurance, this money, and thus, this immortality!"

The central issues of earthly immortality are whether an individual life would have meaning if it went on indefinitely and whether society's needs could sustain an ever-expanding population. The concept of heaven provides a place where the believer may be rewarded with a place, which in many religions, resembles earth (it is a series of mansions, a garden, a city, a party), but has none of the drawbacks of tedium and overpopulation. Perhaps heaven is a consolation to those of us who want most of all continued life *here*, but know deep down that we cannot (and should not) have it.

It's as if we have journeyed all the perilous way to the mouth of the rivers even as we knew that Utnapishtim would decline our prolongevity request. For historical example, Shih-Huang (259–210 BCE) of the Ch'in must have known that elixirs probably wouldn't work, or he wouldn't have commissioned the terra cotta warriors to guard his tomb. Those who live without the awareness that death is always possible operate with less awareness of what existence means, according to philosophers like Kierkegaard and Heidegger. The paradox is that when we live with the understanding that we will die, we often seek to affirm life by mitigating death, which leads to thinking that we might overcome death, which is to live at a lower level of awareness. One can go through the steps of self-awareness and arrive back at the start, which is that death is not a problem for us.

Yet the act of turning to God or Utnapishtim or Science or Creation or Collective Memory to grant us continued, meaningful lives shows that we understand that joining forces with something outside of ourselves may be the only way to save ourselves. In the next chapter, I shall survey the many modes in which a human being may attach himself to other beings, processes, or forces to save himself through merging. Through the merging, the self must be transformed; if it is not transformed, then the merging never wholly took place. The paradox to look out for in this act of joining to a greater power is: how much of the self must one lose to save itself? It is, by the way, the same paradox that attends love, posthumous fame, and Christianity.

CHAPTER SEVEN: MERGING WITH THE ENDURING

Through the infinity of the universe the mind which contemplates it achieves some share in infinity. —Bertrand Russell, from *The Problems of Philosophy*

A god no less, so great you've grown, so swollen . . . feeling all Creation, the whole six days' work, inside yourself, in your pride of strength delighting in — what, I can't imagine. Ecstatically merging with all there is, all being, the earthly creature [is] transcended and forgotten.—Goethe (Martin Greenberg, trans.) *Faust*, Part I: "A Cavern in the Forest"

According to Bertrand Russell (1872–1970 CE), thinking about infinite objects bestows a share of infinity to the mind. Plato's Diotima, as we have seen, also believes that contemplating the enduring Forms offers a taste of immortality. Ansel Adams (1902–1984 CE), on a photography hike in Yosemite, joined his impermanent self to the sublime power of nature. He is said to have found religious comfort in this communion with nature.[1] Believing in and fighting for transcendent causes is believed, by many, to enlarge the self and empower it beyond its own inherent potentials. The soldier who risks his life for his religion, country, ideology, or civilization often does so because the cause, and not his own ephemeral self, has the potential to be more powerful, influential, and enduring. So, like the proverbial downward ball of snow increasing its own stature as it incorporates what used to be "outside" of itself, the human tries to increase his own stature and prospects for continued life by assimilating what he puts in front of himself as an object of thought, belief, or pursuit.

To be clear, merging with the enduring is what we have been talking about since this book began. The lover joins his other half, the fame aspirant abandons himself to the collective memory of civilization, the creative person surrenders his object to the world which continues on without him, the believer subjugates his will to the will of God, and through science or magic the prolongevitor tries to get the earth to be a collaborator, to discard Mother Nature's plan that all shall die and go along with his that he shall live.[2] It is fitting, then, that we conclude with this topic and pick out key moments from our heritage which have set into motion the concept of merging into the infinite. After a few remarks on the concepts of love, fame, creativity, and personal immortality, I look at various key moments in history in which the permanent and immortal was thought to give life to comparatively insignificant, mortal individuals.

LOVE REFINED

Two works which have informed my discussion thus far are the ancient Sumerian epic *Gilgamesh* and the Classical Greek dialogue *The Symposium*. They, as we have seen, both proceed from expectations and assumptions about what love should be. Gilgamesh thinks lovers should be faithful forever (excepting himself). Socrates and Diotima agree that love is much more than finding one's other half: it is finding one's kinship with the eternal Forms. Gilgamesh's expectations of love initiate a series of events that culminate in his futile search for lasting earthly life. Plato's placement, in the *Symposium*, of Alcibiades's encounter with Socrates to elucidate that Socrates did not think much of the cave of earthly love and fleshy pleasure. Alcibiades, the story goes, pursues a sexual encounter with Socrates after a night of drinking. Socrates turns him down. Finding no delight in the delights that others prize and pursue, Socrates shows that the primary love worth seeking is that which merges the individual with the undying Forms. People die and pleasures do not last; so why love them? For a love that really lasts, one must love a thing that lasts. For Diotima, the Forms are essentially the only Other that secure the lastingness that Gilgamesh demands from Ishtar, and our language (e.g., "I will love you forever and ever") indicates that we consider ideal.

In Plato's *Symposium*, prior to Socrates's outlining Diotima's theory of love, we had been invited to consider the Other Half theory of love proffered by Aristophanes. Aristophanes defends the view that we seek each other because in our most natural state, before offending Zeus, we were joined together as one substance. These more powerful humans planned mutiny against the Olympian gods. To prevent further insolence, Zeus wanted to debilitate the human race. After a series of experiments, Zeus settled on having us be halves of what we were so that we'd lose our power to challenge his dominance. But being half of what we should be puts us on an incessant search to become whole again:

> By the mutual embraces of man and woman they [humans] might breed, and the race might continue; . . . so ancient is the desire of one another which is implanted in us, reuniting our original nature, making one of two, and healing the state of man. Each of us when separated, having one side only, like a flat fish, is but the indenture of a man, and he is always looking for his other half.[3]

On Aristophanes's view, love is primarily physical and procreative. This view is set into high relief by Diotima's view that love should be understood as primarily mental. For her, the Forms are a kind of immortal dwelling for the lover. The Forms grant those who contemplates them a share of their infinity. One may quite readily see a corollary with lovers of the divine. By loving God, we hope to dwell with Him: on earth, with prayer, and in heaven, upon death.

What are we to make of the trade deficit incurred by dwelling in God's domain? In the case of loving God (or loving Forms), the lover seems to get more than he gives. He gains immortality and knowledge. He might praise God or delight in the Forms, but both exist in their glory, whether the individual joins them or not. "You have no need of our praise, yet our desire to thank you is itself your gift: our prayer of thanksgiving adds nothing to your greatness" may be heard in Catholic masses all around the world.

Compared to loving God and gaining what he can grant, loving material things is not worth our attention. St. Augustine (354–430 CE) writes in his *Confessions* of the days, prior to his saintly days, when he loved the world of the flesh and ignored his highest, spiritual identity, which led him to live a self-inflicted unfulfilling existence with the impermanent and transient. He wasted his time dwelling with those things that were alien to his spiritual nature and destiny. He came around to see, through Christianity and Platonism, that one should forsake the items of this world and love the permanent. Love of God trumps all other love.

One should not underestimate that being loved by God is perhaps more important as loving God when it comes to gaining immortality from the relation. If not for God's love for us, especially in the Abrahamic religions, then the individual is helpless against death. The Christian verse is explicit: "For God so loved the world that He gave His only begotten Son, that whosoever believeth in Him should not perish, but have eternal life."[4] The message is unequivocal: we perish without God's love for us. This precept of faith reverberates all the more when we contrast it with fate promised by Epicurus, Lucretius, Epictetus, and Aurelius: death is nothingness.

Even for the lover of God death may be nothingness. By this, I mean that while we are dead, we are nothing. Consider the Christian resurrection. Many believe in a "resurrection of the dead," which restores the life lost by death. This belief affirms that death is nothingness, but resurrection saves us from that state. It is not a denial of death and its powers, but rather a belief that death can be overcome through God's love. This resurrection, whether spiritual or physical, provides solace to the weary who recognize the mortal truth in both *Ecclesiastes* and Marcus Aurelius. When one is loved by a God capable of doing anything, one could come out of death alive. If God gave us life from nothingness the first time, can't we hope He'll do it again? Blaise Pascal (1623–1662 CE) puts it well:

What reason do atheists have to say that one cannot rise from the dead? Which
is the more difficult, to be born or to be reborn? That that which has never existed should exist, or that that which existed should exist again?[5]

We can love God all we want and try to attach ourselves to His eternality, but if
the love is unrequited, it will be as if we never loved Him at all. He might deny
us His love and He might deny us the immortality we seek.

So, whether attaching ourselves to another half to bring forth new physical
life, or to a Form to achieve a taste of immortal truth, or to a God who grants us
continued life, love is essentially a merging into an object beyond ourselves with
the capability to enlarge ourselves, to empower ourselves to do what we could
not do alone.

FAME'S DEPENDENCIES

Fame aspirants also, potentially, draw their continued life from others. The
collective memory of others is a prerequisite for fame. Without memory, fame is
impossible. With trust, fame seekers entrust their desires to be remembered onto
others, who they may not even know. Unlike the religious person who relies on
and praises the divine for granting continued life, the fame-seeker relies on future humans, yet considers *herself worthy of the praise*. Louis XIV, who thought
that his fame was the most precious thing on earth, was not out to praise the
people who recall his image and deeds. They were pawns, mostly forgettable
pawns, but what an important role these pawns played in calling Louis to mind.

The relationship between the deceased famous person and the collective
memory of the living, though, is a symbiotic one. The living must remember the
dead for fame to persist, and so, the famous person relies on the living. However, at the same time he relies on them to remember him, his fame is itself a
kind of posthumous control over the living. His name and deeds are there to be
summoned and they command the attention of the living that memorialize him.
If you take a person like Muhammad, the founder of Islam, and consider his
fame, the paradox is readily seen. Without the living to continue his faith and
read the *Koran* transmitted through him, he is forgotten: the living have the
power in this regard. Yet, Muhammad stands out as the last of the prophets and
his memory directly influences millions of people: the deceased has power. If
his image is treated with disrespect, the ones remembering him take notice.
Some take action. The merging of the famous with the collective memory, then,
also occurs conversely insofar as the collectivity receives its identity from the
famous. Fame enlarges "the remembered," giving the famous person a continued mode of life (as memory) and defines "the ones remembering," giving that
community a shared commonality.[6]

CREATIVITY'S ALLIANCES

The creative person wishes his product or idea to last for future people to engage with, and ultimately, to remember the creator. He hopes for an enduring universe to sustain his product's existence. In fact, he depends on it.

For thought's sake, imagine that Leonardo Da Vinci knew his *Last Supper* experimental fresco technique would lessen the durability of the final product. As we know, his painting over the dry wall with tempera led to his product losing its form and pigment in many places. Let's suppose that he could have known that this technique would shorten the life of his painting to a decade or two. He may even with this hypothetical foresight have decided to create it in the experimental way regardless, because he balanced his need to make his best possible work with his desire to have it last. Obviously all it needed was two decades of existence in its completed and undeteriorated state.[7] This was enough to secure not only fame for the work, ensuring (as well as fame can) that future individuals will have interest in the work, but also critical acclaim and admiration. Supposing, then, that Da Vinci knew his work would not last in optimal form, he may have recognized that creating the best possible object would secure its place in the future well enough, even if that best possible object was not in its best possible form for long. Architects and city planners also make trade-offs between the ideal work and the practicalities affecting durability.

Fame and creative legacy thus become entangled when the work achieves fame even though the artifact itself is diminished (or even annihilated). When the work is there, it can stand for the artist. When the fame is there, the living may very well dedicate their careers to preserving the artifact (e.g., Da Vinci's *Last Supper*) or even rediscovering a work (e.g., Da Vinci's *Battle of Anghiari*). The artifact can spawn fame and fame kindles motivation to uncover legacy. Both fame and creative legacy require the reliance of the individual upon others: the persistence of a memory or the continuation of a stable universe.

RELIGIONS' SUCCESSES

Miguel de Unamuno (1864–1936 CE) wrote in his philosophical treatise *The Tragic Sense of Life* that the Catholic Church exists to respond to the terror of our impending deaths.[8] This idea also surfaces in a character from his short story, *San Manuel Bueno, Martyr*. Don Manuel, himself a priest, does not believe in an afterlife, and yet he acknowledges, by his actions, the importance of the Church's function to help people to "die well."[9] Catholic Christianity is far from the only religion that provides answers for what is to come after death, thus making death more bearable.

When we think about religious worldviews, especially the five world religions, we recognize that even they all place some premium on a well-lived life on earth. The Hindu must live well now to attain a satisfactory next life, the Buddhist must work within the parameters of this life to liberate himself from attachments, the Jew must uphold the covenant with Yahweh, the Muslim must follow the precepts of almsgiving and justice to make it to the garden of paradise, and even Jesus Christ recognized that our time on earth is a precious time in which good deeds must be done: "I must work the works of him that sent me, whilst it is day: the night cometh, when no man can work"[10] Although spiritual aspirations and alliances must take place while one is *on* earth, these cannot be *of the* earth, since earth itself does not offer permanence.

Some who worship Mother Earth may believe that they will live on through the continuation of the planet. But as we have seen at the end of chapter three (on fame), the universe and its earth will not last forever. Merging with the earth will (likely) buy one's molecules time after one has died, but that time is destined to run out even if one does not know the precise hour. Some Christians expect to "inherit the earth"[11] in a literal sense, but even they cannot ally themselves *with the earth* to attain immortality. They inherit the earth precisely by turning from the earth and towards God and others. Even the Eastern faiths of Hinduism and Buddhism, with less personalized afterlives, can bring comfort. Reuniting with Brahman and escaping a life of suffering are happy thoughts. Whether Eastern or Western, the individual who seeks spiritual prolongevity must transcend himself and this life to join a higher reality, or depend on a higher reality to help the transcendence occur.

That any given individual human lives now, intact with his self-consciousness, is a statistical miracle, why not count on another life?[12] We didn't ask for the statistical miracle that we're here *now*. We do ask for continued life. Why couldn't God help out an individual hoping for a tomorrow? We would do it ourselves if we could. In fact, we try for it, in any way we can (e.g., love, fame, creativity). Some attempt experimental treatments and even freeze themselves to bring them closer to Methuselah's record of life.

Living our continued life in the spiritual world, since it is beyond our control, requires a leap of faith and a reliance on a being unseen. The Christian believes we get our eternal life by living in the light of God. Heaven is possible because God secures it. The Muslim believes the same, and like the Christian, believes that God secures it and determines who will have access to it. There is no sneaking into heaven. Even the Hindu or Buddhist, without a personal God, still has to depend on an ontological order and playing by the way it's set up to gain *moksha*, or release, from this life.

In all cases of spiritual immortality, the believer requires the Other (the divine or an ambassador of the divine) to grant continued life, freedom from death, and a life worth continuing. As fame and creative legacy overlap, religious belief overlaps with love. The believer depends on God's love.

EARTHLY IMMORTALITY IN REALITY

The allure of prolonging one's life on earth, however, even for the religious person, is strong and we must not deny its pull on us. Most of us like life and want it to continue, thinking life will be better in the future; e.g., we'll be in better shape, we'll have more money, we'll have more time in the day to do the things we love. However unwittingly, we ally ourselves with things of the earth in hopes to give ourselves a better future.

Alliances with the earth and worldly concerns can be much like seeking love. We seek the other (in this case education, employment, family ties, etc.) and, in so doing, we assume a future as we serve ourselves and our interests. It is enlarging ourselves through seeking something outside of ourselves. Prolongevity is a clinging to the things of this life to acquire a worthwhile future. That forward-looking attitude is the feeling of immortality described in chapter one and throughout this book.

Subsequent sections of this chapter will examine historical and philosophical themes of merging with the immortal to the supposed benefit of mortal humans.

THEME ONE: ALLIANCES WITH THE DIVINE AND HUMAN JUSTICE

We look back to Babylon, to an era and place where a human being was attempting to bring order to a region with an already lengthy history of war and strife. Hammurabi (r. 1792–1750 BCE) was ruler of Babylon. The *Gilgamesh* epic produced in that region was already one-thousand-years-old. Hammurabi, perhaps being a clever politician or perhaps truly believing a god revealed laws to him, allied himself with the immortal divinity of Shamash to establish, justify, and preserve laws of human justice. Justice is, of course, not easily defined. Is it giving to each their due? Is it an equitable distribution of rights and resources? Is it the equitable application of fair procedures (as opposed to outcomes)? Whatever our best understandings of justice, we note that justice has something to do with how we relate to other human beings. It is a horizontal relationship: it is between fellow humans. So, justice must cover our responsibilities to and expectations of each other. This horizontal relationship is the virtue of acting properly towards other human beings. Justice stands in contrast to the vertical relationship we may have with superior beings (piety) or lower life forms (fiduciary).

With *Hammurabi's Code*, a vertical relationship with an immortal god backs up his proclamations of the horizontal relationships of human justice. It justifies his justice. A stele inscribed with Hammurabi's famous law code, found today at the Louvre in Paris, features a relief of the god Shamash giving the laws to Hammurabi.

Hammurabi derives two benefits from allying himself (and his laws) with the divine. These have much to do with concepts of immortality. First, humans prove more motivated to follow the law if they come from, or at the very least, are endorsed by, a source that will not die. Hammurabi's subjects would be more likely to follow the code if it originated at the level of the gods. The gods will be around to see to it that lawbreakers get their due. So, it is likely that, on balance, people would be more inclined to take them seriously since they came from on high. Hammurabi must have been astute to recognize another tangible benefit of sharing the lawmaker-credit with Shamash.

The second benefit of giving credit to the divine is that Hammurabi reserves his place of privilege in the cosmic hierarchy of gods and humans by this act. He talks to the god. The god talks to him and commands him "to make justice appear in the land." The god trusts in Hammurabi to act on his behalf. Hammurabi becomes chosen, anointed; a proxy for the god. So, even as he ascribes the authorship credits to Shamash, he gains "political capital" and esteem, since he is an *associate* of Shamash. Turning again to the Louvre stele, we notice that these remarks are consistent with the Hammurabi portrayed in the relief. He appears as one conferencing with the god, yet the more largely depicted god appears the primary authority on his throne. The delicate balance between the authority of Hammurabi and his service to the god is achieved by the artist.

When one thinks of the Judaic Ten Commandments enumerated in *Exodus*, one is struck by a similar theme. God, it may be said, commands Moses, to make justice appear. In fact, seventy percent of the laws given to Moses (commandments four through ten) have to do with horizontal relationships between humans whereas the other three govern their vertical dealings with God.[13] The message is clear from these early sources of law: people don't sketch the precepts of justice. Justice is commanded with the force and authority of God. Moreover, the laws of justice do not change because their author (God) always exists. The laws of justice need to be heeded at all times because God always exists. These lawgivers, Hammurabi and Moses, allied themselves with immortal gods, and they expected their people to do the same.

Like Hammurabi and Moses, Thomas Jefferson (1743–1826 CE) famously links the revolutionary cause in America to the eternal God's granting of rights and human duties. Moreover, it is our duty to dissolve those human institutions in conflict with God's will:

> We hold these truths to be self-evident, that all men are created equal, that they are endowed by their Creator with certain unalienable Rights, that among these are Life, Liberty and the pursuit of Happiness. — That to secure these rights, Governments are instituted among Men, deriving their just powers from the consent of the governed, — That whenever any Form of Government becomes destructive of these ends, it is the Right of the People to alter or to abolish it, and to institute new Government, laying its foundation on such principles and organizing its powers in such form, as to them shall seem most likely to effect their Safety and Happiness.[14]

The Creator assigns the principles of justice, and it is up to the people to see to it that they are upheld (just like it is up to Hammurabi to be the steward of justice). Like Hammurabi and Moses, Jefferson and his disciples conceived God to be an enduring force that has certain preferences for how life is to be lived on earth. It is up to us to live up to them.

The feeling that justice derives from God (Divine Command Theory) rather than humans is unsettling to many in our present age. Any appeal to a divinity to justify public policy and law is not easily defended by proponents. We trust our collective reason to establish justice, and religion is too often used to justify abuses of morality and justice. There is also a philosophical problem with God being the founder and sustainer of justice. If God defines justice and God can do anything (i.e., if God is omnipotent), then why can't God change about what is just and unjust? If God lives forever, then he *can* change his mind at any point in time for the whole of history. Actions, *in themselves*, are neither just nor unjust so long as their moral status is wholly fastened to the will of God. But, wouldn't we all agree that there is something inherently unjust about murdering an innocent person? If God gives actions their moral status as just or unjust, we have to maintain the possibility that God could simply give murder a 'just' rating rather than an 'unjust' rating. To this, it could be argued that God is immutable. He doesn't change, and therefore, he doesn't change his will. Yet even with an immutable God who *does* not change his will, he *could* still change his will. If he couldn't, then he wouldn't be all-powerful and, therefore, wouldn't be God. Suffice it to say that the Hammurabi or Moses of today would have considerable difficulty winning support in a modern democratic state or in academia.

Another problem with the Divine Command Theory is whether we can be certain that we know that the moral law has its source in the divine. How can we distinguish between the decrees of a king, like Hammurabi and the decrees of God, especially when the decrees of God are issued through the king? Plato explores the relationship between the divine and the moral law in his *Euthyphro*, written one thousand years after the events in *Exodus*. The *Euthyphro* conclusions challenge the assumptions that we can know the will of God, that we would be able to apply it even if we knew it, and that it might change at any time given the flexibility for a God to change His mind. Of course, the eternal rule of law is not equal to the immortal Self. Yet these examples from early history show the human inclination to rest its projects on the strength of the eternal and, consequently, to draw on the force of immortality to give human projects power and durability. This tactic will soon be used to give the Self the property of immortality previously reserved for projects such as justice and obedience.

THEME TWO: TOMBS AND TRUST IN THE EARTH'S LONGEVITY

In his September 18, 2001 speech, President George W. Bush declared that Islamo-Fascism would "take its rightful place in history's unmarked grave of discarded lies." The unmarked grave represents the forgotten, the uncared for, and those not taken seriously. "Our existence does not have any significance for the future" is what the unmarked grave expresses. If one goes to Washington D.C.'s tomb of the Unknown Soldier, the spectator witnesses a guarded tomb in which the unidentified is remembered, is cared about, and is taken seriously.

The device of the Unknown Soldier burial place is widely used in many countries across the globe. Why?

Let us first think about the marked grave site. The marked grave site is not only a site of respect, but it becomes a space that individuates the individual, and is not occupied by another. The grave stone, or stele as was the case in earlier centuries, is a lasting (I have learned better than to say "permanent") monument placed at a site. The soul is not part of the terrestrial world, but the human remains remain (even if they become dust) and the marker remains. And like a creative artifact, the marked grave site prompts reflection about the interred's existence. In this profound sense, then, we are relying on the universe's stability and partitioning off a piece of it for ourselves. And, why not? We were granted to interact with it while we were alive. We were its molecules. We breathed its air and moved its soil and water to facilitate our life on the planet.

To not have a marked gravesite is to be forgotten, cast aside, unacknowledged, unappreciated, and in sum, one who did not make enough of an impact.

What about the tombs of the Unknowns, then? They are not marked, but guarded, respected, and visited. They extend to other unidentified fallen soldiers and pay them acknowledgement and posthumous praise. They boost the reputation[15] of the anonymous individual interred (and the individuals referred to by extension) more than an ordinary marked grave could have done.

It is worth considering that news outlets reported that the remains in occupying the Unknown tomb at Arlington National Cemetery are those of Michael Joseph Blassie, whose plane was shot down in Vietnam (1972). Blassie's mother said that she wanted her son to have his own marked grave.[16] Yet, out of the 300,000 graves at Arlington, the tomb of the Unknown is widely considered to be the most sacrosanct. With this case we see two powerful forces coming together: (1) the individual as part of an enduring receives more power from joining with it, and (2) the individual has his individuality threatened by losing itself in the enduring. After all, one can not be an Unknown soldier and at the same time have an accurately marked grave. One would have to join the other 300,000 individuals and, almost certainly, get less attention.

THEME THREE: GREEK PRESOCRATIC IMMORTALITY

Presocratic philosophers, philosophers before Socrates (469–399 BCE), found immortality in the elements, the natural world, and natural processes. The world is as it is not because of some whim of an undying god, but because undying principles and processes are at work. These principles and processes are predictable, and thus must transcend contingencies of time and place. By uniting the human mind with these immortalities of scientific principles and processes, the individual eventually came to transcend itself. The story of Greek philosophy begins with naturalism and ends with humanism.

Thales (c. 585 BCE) believed that the material underpinning of the natural world is water. The element water was the unchanging substance that could explain all diversity in the cosmos. But Thales did not make much of a case as to *how* water appears as different things. In other words, Thales does not argue for any *undying ordering process* which acts upon water to change it into rocks, earth, and insects. Thales's successor Anaximander (ca. 610–546 BCE) introduces the first principle of <apeiron>[17], usually translated as "the boundless," to preside over the transformations of the elements. Water, earth, air, and fire change into one another by the operation of <apeiron>. Water may change into earth, but the principle even more basic than that, <apeiron>, *remains continuous and unceasing*. Anaximenes (c. 546 BCE) declared the ultimate material principle to be air, but also specified an *unceasing* process by which air is transformed into the diversity we observe. Anaximenes's process had to do with air becoming more dense (condensation) or less dense (rarefaction). Importantly, neither air nor the process by which air was transformed into the other elements was dependent upon the fiat of the gods. Immortality was to be found in the realm of the natural rather than the supernatural. Anaximenes:

> Attributed all the causes of things to infinite, and did not deny that there were gods, or pass them over in silence; yet he believed not the air was made by them, but that they arose from air.[18]

The questions of these earliest of philosophers were undoubtedly scientific. Their answers, though, do presuppose a leap from the observable experience of the plural, temporary, and changing to the reasoned trust in the basic, lasting, and permanent. Therefore, we must understand their assumptions as a search for the mode of immortality that they believed must exist to make observations trustworthy and repeatable from one moment to the next. Stability is important for the observant scientist.

The philosophies of other Presocratics, Parmenides (ca. 570–478 BCE) and Heraclitus (c. 500 BCE), are sometimes regarded as inconsistent. Parmenides argued that being (i.e., what exists) never changes. Being is therefore immortal. Heraclitus argued that being is always changing. Being is therefore never the same from one moment to the next. In fact, what exists passes away and what does not exist comes to be. Being itself is in constant flux for Heraclitus. From one moment to the next, it changes. He went so far as to say that we never step into the same river twice, indicating that both the "river" and the "we" have changed. We might be led to think that Parmenides is the immortalist and Heraclitus is the anti-immortalist. The truth is that each philosopher affirmed a significant, albeit different, concept of immortality. Parmenides affirmed that what exists always exists, never changes, and cannot be divided. This is the immortality of substance. Heraclitus affirmed that the process of constant change always exists and never changes. This is the immortality of process. If the process itself were subject to change or cessation, Heraclitus's philosophy itself would change. It would not explain the process as it is now, but as it was at some previous moment. His philosophy would lose all its explanatory significance.

Parmenides and Heraclitus had compatible programs of thought, at least in terms of some of their basic assumptions. Yet philosophers after them wanted to do more than understand that the two programs could coexist: they wanted to *reconcile* them. The two had seemingly disparate theses about stability and change, and yet each thesis could be observed in the real world. Parmenides's thought that being remains the same is verified by our ability to recognize someone we haven't seen in twenty years, but Heraclitus's thought that being is in constant flux is verified by our ability to recognize that the very same person we identified later now has graying hair, a pot belly, and a twenty year bank of memories since we've last seen them. They seem to have stayed the same insofar as we can recognize them (Parmenides), but they appear different (Heraclitus).

The atomists, such as Democritus (460–370 BCE), argued that the world is made up of tiny, indestructible, and indivisible atoms. In this claim, they remained faithful to Parmenides. Yet, they argued that these atoms were indeed in a constant state of flux because they were constantly bumping into one another, creating new composites. So, in this atomist claim, the atomists also remained faithful to Heraclitus. *Both the immortalities of being and process were acknowledged.* This is, of course, not what one would consider a triumph of the individual ego insofar as these concepts of immortality do not help us know whether we live forever or die into nonexistence. But they do help make science possible. We can study the world because *what we are studying* (i.e., being) will not change in the middle of our experiments. We can apply testing and *consistent processes* such as the scientific method because we have confidence that the processes will be as dependable now as they were in the past.

Equipped with the conception of a stable universe and the early scientific method emphasizing observation and human reason, the scientist can find communion with the material world. The immortality of this other, the universe, affects the immortality prospects for the Self's being remembered, having its work continue to exist, and whether future persons will pray for its soul or visit its gravesite.

THEME FOUR: HUMANISM: THE IMMORTALITY OF COLLECTIVE BEING

The individual may seek to merge itself with the human spirit, which Ludwig Feuerbach (1804–1872 CE) thought to be the only immortality attainable:

> Your belief in immortality is a true belief only when it is a belief in the infinity of the Spirit and in the everlasting youth of humanity, in the inexhaustible love and creative power of Spirit, in its eternally unfolding itself into new individuals out of the womb of its plenitude and granting new beings for glorification, enjoyment, and contemplation of itself.[19]

Over 2500 years before Feuerbach, Greek artists collectively celebrated the human form and, by extension, the human spirit. Eventually, the Greek philosophers caught on. It is indeed interesting to note that it was the philosophers who had to catch up to the humanistic emphasis of the artists rather than the other way around. While the philosophers were looking at the empirical world in search of immortal being and immortal process, the artists were looking inward to the enduring human spirit.

Back to the artists: the sculptural record left to us shows that the Archaic Greeks set artists on course to triumphantly exalt the human. Thus, they began the most serious attempt hitherto to bring out the timeless and undying beauty of what might be called the human spirit. Even within the Archaic style (approx. 600–480 BCE), a progression is readily seen. Such preclassical sculpture is an informative slideshow of attempts to reveal the eternal. I shall give highlights from that important progression, but first, for contrast, let us recall that realism is of value to different communities for different reasons. For example, the Egyptian artists were dedicated to a brand of realism, the realistic portrayal of this or that individual, and they were faithful even to the detail of imperfections. The reason for their dedication to realism is that accurate portrayal was important for the soul recognizing its tomb. Ramses II (1279–1213 BCE) provides a well-known example of this. His nose was quite distinguishable and pronounced. So, both his artists and his morticians made significant efforts to conserve that idiosyncratic nose.

Another community might also value realism for a different, less spiritual reason. The Greeks were quite concerned with this world. They were comfortable in it. Without a vivid concept of a worthwhile afterlife, Greeks treasured their stories and bodies alike. Artists were increasingly expected to produce works mirroring earthly life itself. They were expected to portray realistic stances, glances, and musculature. Yet, for the Greeks, accurate portrayal gave way to idealization. For them, realism was the path to idealism.

Even the early Archaic subjects of the sculptures were not usually the common, randomized man *as he was* (as in the pharaoh Ramses II's case), but rather well-built and beautiful and youthful subjects. Youthful subjects were the models for the kourai. Early on, these "cherry-picked" subjects were made to stand in rigid but dignified postures. With left foot stepping forward, the *Kouros from Sounion* (ca. 615–590 BCE) and the *New York Kouros* (ca. 615–590 BCE) resemble each other. Apart from their suggested movements, both kourai are fixed and almost tense. The dignified positions restrained the expression of true youthful exuberance. But in time the artists portrayed similar subjects stepping forward in more convincing poses and casting warmer smiles as if in waiting for a photographer to shoot a photo. For example, the *Ptoon Kouros* (ca. 540–520 BCE) already boasts of a more relaxed stance, a smile, and increased vitality. In less than one hundred years, the progression to the immortal human spirit was well under way.

A similar progression may be noted when comparing the female *Auxerre Kore* (675–600 BCE) to the *Peplos Kore* (535–530 BCE). The *Peplos Kore* is much more realistic, elastic, warm, and detailed (for example, see her hair); she is also more ideal. Her disposition, smile, and figure approach the ideal. Through a mixing of realism and idealism, the Greek sculptor was beginning to reveal the living spirit of not only this or that person, but of all humanity.

It is at this point that we may bring up a paradox in this early Greek world-view. One would think that by paying more attention to the details of a subject's stance, posture, facial expressions, musculature, and the like, artists would end up with a more realistic product than if they forced each subject to conform to an already worked out caste of stance and form. In an important sense, this observation is true. The Archaic Greeks, in time, successfully released their subjects from the confining and unrealistic molds of the standardized poses. And it is true that in releasing the subject from clichéd positioning, observation of detail became emphasized.

However, there are two important senses in which this point of Greek realism is misleading. We must not mistake realism for lack of transcendence, for lack of idealism. First, the purpose of the Greek realism was not so much to display the idiosyncrasies of the individual as an artist working in Egypt would have it. Personality cannot shine through fully as long as there are formulas of design to be followed. Greek realism was aimed at revealing how the human body, in general, *could be* when fit in physique and relaxed in stance. Their realism aimed at revealing the ideal, and the ideal must be understood as the ideal human.

Secondly, the subjects for the Greek realists do not seem to be taken from the population in general. The overwhelming majority of subjects are taken from a demographic of beautiful subjects aged between fifteen and twenty one. The selective sample of vibrant human beings in peak shape expresses ideal and transcendent human characteristics. Athletes may lose their physique or competing prowess, but the ideal physique remains unchanging and undying. In Greek sculpture, we have seen a sharp development of the concepts of ceaseless ideal human characteristics, which transcend any one human being's temporary possession of them.

So, in summary, that some human beings were shown how they were, the entire group of human beings was referred to. In ethics, there is often a great divide between what is and what should be. In the progression of early Greek sculpture, the divide between the *is* and the *should be*, the real and the ideal, was purposely narrowed by talented artists who assuredly brought objects into being which closely resembled their own ideals of how a human should be.

THEME FIVE: CLASSICAL GREECE:
MERGING THE INDIVIDUAL WITH THE ENDURING UNIVERSE AND
HUMANISM

The Classical period in Greece begins in the decades immediately preceding their 480 BCE victory over the Persians. This period was Athens's finest hour. Athenian drama, architecture, politics, prosperity, and philosophy were simply unrivaled by any previous civilization or concurrent civilization. Within that one-hundred-year period, one may find concepts of the immortal which continue to influence present day western culture and rhetoric.

We may begin by noting, along with Victor Davis Hanson, the transcendence of freedom.[20] In 490 BCE, when the Persian Empire sought to conquer the Greeks, the Greek city-states were able create an alliance and fight off the threat. And why were the Greeks capable of putting aside their differences and uniting against the wealthy and centralized power with a nearly global reach? The transcendence of freedom. When one believes they are fighting on behalf of an idea larger than themselves and larger than their epoch, they fight harder than those who fight for kings, aristocrats, and priests.[21] Athenian life was worth defending, and freedom is a much bigger idea than any individual.

Athens, Sparta, and the Greek alliance put aside internal differences and repelled the Persian attackers, but not without human and infrastructure losses. The acropolis of Athens was utterly destroyed by Xerxes's Persian army. After a moratorium on building on the site (to honor the fallen), the Athenians turned their attention to rebuilding their city.

The *Parthenon* (i.e., the temple dedicated to Athena) was, and still is, seen as the centerpiece of the new and glorious Athenian acropolis. What kind of temple do you build for a deity who will never die and whose faithfulness to the future of the city-state is likewise undying? It seems fitting to have your design reflect immortality. The design that Pericles (r. 461–429 BCE), longtime elected leader of Athens, chose for the *Parthenon* (a temple dedicated to Athena) mirrored the philosophy of Pythagoras, complete with his immortal mathematical concepts. The Doric Order *Parthenon* reflects what Greeks considered divine proportions. Its pediments and friezes were sculpted in a style, which glorified the struggles of a free people who invested their lives in the service of freedom itself. Both its architecture and its sculpture converge in service not only to the gods, but to civic esteem and confidence in a political system and a way of life.

When we left the story of philosophy last, we were discussing the concepts of immortality as material and process. Pythagoras (571–497 BCE) subtly weighs in on the issue by ignoring questions of material reality and concentrating on issues of pure, formal existence, which he believed was immaterial numbers. The Pythagorean concentration would shape the *Parthenon's* architectural design. Here is how.

For Pythagoras, the religious leader, the soul is immortal. It exists even after the body is dead: it transmigrates to another body. But while the soul inhabits a body, the body's concerns ought not to be the soul's concerns. Why should it waste its time in the ever-changing and unstable world of the senses when it could contemplate the everlasting and stable? The immortal soul should contemplate something that is most like itself in its immortality: numbers. Numbers do not die or pass away. Numbers reveal themselves in objects, but are not destroyed by the object's destruction. For example, if one holds up a right triangle cut out of paper, the Pythagorean Theorem (the square of the hypotenuse of a right-angled triangle is equal to the sum of the squares other sides) may be applied to that triangle. Now, suppose I burn the paper triangle to ashes; the triangle is gone, but the theorem remains. Suppose even that I somehow disposed of every right triangle in the universe, would not the theorem still hold true? It is immortal. In fact, if all rational beings capable of knowing the Pythagorean Theorem disappeared, wouldn't the Theorem still hold true? Using the terminology that subsequent philosophers would later adopt, Pythagoras believed that the Form is true reality which exists forever and the matter is not true reality, since it is continuously subject to change. So, mathematics is primary to sensible reality, but it may be exhibited within that sensible reality.

Pythagoras believed that mathematical harmony is present in musical harmony as well. If one cuts the length of a string in half, the octave harmony will be heard. If one cuts it in half and compares it with a string cut in thirds, one will hear the fifth harmony. One may also compare a string cut in thirds to a string quartered, in that case, a fourth harmony is heard. The octave, fourth, and fifth harmony together makes a full sounding major chord, pleasing to the ears. Pythagoras believed that the seven different sounds of the scale are pleasing because they are a faithful translation of the formal, mathematical, and eternal order of the universe.

Pythagoras and his followers believed that this musical order reflected the celestial order. Pythagoras's views connecting music, proportion, and the cosmos are clearly expressed by the Roman Cicero (106–43 BCE):

> This uppermost sphere of the heavens bearing the stars, since it revolves at greater speed, moves apace with notes of highest pitch, while that one of the moon, the lowest, gives out the lowest tones; for the earth, ninth of the spheres, remains without motion in its fixed place in the centre of the universe. But the other eight spheres, two of which move at the same rate [Mercury and Venus], send out seven different sounds, — that number which is the key of almost anything.[22]

We may, then, access the divine order through music because the mathematical properties of music and harmony are the same as those underpinning the cosmos.

Athena, being the goddess of Reason, is a perfect candidate to receive a temple reflecting the knowable, formal, mathematical, and immortal order of the universe. Ictinus and Callicrates designed their temple to Athena according to the musical octave (1:2), a symmetry celebrated by Pythagoras as expressing the rational order of the universe. Alliance with the gods is not far away. Before we examine that leap, let us look at humanistic impulses which take shape without positing reliance on the gods or God.

HUMANISM WITHOUT GOD

Classical Athenians saw many goods flowing into their imperial city in the Periclean golden age. Among the imports were Sophists. These men walked the streets of the Athenian agora at the same time as the Athenian born Socrates. The Sophists were a group of philosophers united in their confining themselves to subject matters of getting along in the world, keeping distance from any lofty concepts of immortal being, processes, Forms, gods, or even truth that occupied other philosophers of their day. Ironically, their indifference to or assault of these lofty concepts was an implicit support of faith in the enduring spirit and worth of the human, which is not the most tangible of subjects. Critias (ca. 460–403 BCE) challenged the gods' existence and, *a fortiori*, their immortality when he stated:

> As the laws did hold men back from deeds of open violence, but still such deeds were done in secret, — then as I maintain, some shrewd man first, a man in counsel wise, discovered unto men the fear of gods, thereby to frighten sinners should they sin even secretly in deed, or word, or thought. Hence, was it that he brought in Deity.[23]

Critias thus defends the view that the concept of immortal gods assists the laws in governing human behavior. Without the gods and their promises of punishment and reward, humans might transgress the laws in secret. He does not claim that the laws themselves were derived from divine sources as Hammurabi did. But, the "shrewd" ruler's intent is the same in both cases: to use the supernatural as a political instrument to ensure obedience. Hammurabi draws upon the powerful and deathless gods to compel compliance to his code; Critias would characterize Hammurabi's "Shamash told me to give these laws" tactic as calculated political expediency. Divine inspiration, Critias thought, is an orchestrated illusion.

Protagoras (ca. 490–420 BCE) is remembered as a staunch humanist. He famously declared, "Man is the measure of all things." On the subject of the gods, Protagoras was not as bold as Critias who claimed to know all about the gods (namely, that there are none!), Protagoras admitted that he knew not whether the gods exist, since life is short and the subject, theology, is obscure. Critias was an atheist, Protagoras was an agnostic. The atheist believes that the gods do not exist. The agnostic, in theory and etymology, has not made up his mind either way. Rather than turning to human conventions to explain or learn from the gods in the manner that later Scholastic philosophers would (c. 1200s

CE), Protagoras thought that we should turn to human conventions to solve practical problems.

Perhaps the art and democracy of Athens inspired his thoughts. The artists, especially the sculptors, of his day had the benefit of over two hundred years of innovation. They learned how to produce lifelike, athletic, beautiful, and sometimes daring portrayals of humans and gods. In many causes, the humans and gods could hardly be distinguished from one another. The de-pedistalization of the gods and the simultaneous pedistalization of the ideal human being created the effect and sentiment that humans could shape their present world as the Olympian gods had shaped it in the poets' writings. Citizens were shaping public policy as never before. Citizens created a public sphere worth living in. Society, greater than any individual within it, was in fact seen as the precondition for all individuals' happiness. As Aristotle (384–322 BCE) wrote, "Man is by nature a political animal . . . [and] when separated from law and justice, he is worst of all."[24] The individual is part of the whole, which, somewhat inexplicably, is greater than the sum of its parts.

Why wouldn't Man, the collective Whole, be the measure of all things? They couldn't know if the gods exist or not, but each day the Athenians witnessed the highest quality art and an open, democratic society, based on the notion that human ideas can solve problems. Sophocles (496–406 BCE) captures the spirit Protagoras when he writes in *Antigone*, "Wonders are many but none is more wonderful than man." In ignoring the religious question of immortality, Protagoras embraces the artists' quest to celebrate a humanistic immortality. In humanism, the individual merges not with the spirit of God, but with the human spirit.

PLATO AND IDEALISM

Born just a few years after the *Parthenon* was completed, Plato (427–347 BCE) is considered the foremost proponent of Formalism, the belief that there are immaterial and eternal Forms which underpin all other sorts of experience, particularly our experiences of the material world.

Plato's commitment to Idealism was unwavering. Idealism, for Plato, refers to the existence of transcendent, immaterial, and eternal concepts by which all earthly substances obtain their existences and definitions (essences). The philosopher, the one who loves wisdom recognizes that goodness is a standard which is not dependent upon any instantiation of it. "Goodness" the idea is not dependent upon "good" acts. If there were no good acts, there would still be goodness. In this, Plato's Idealism recalls the reasoning of Pythagoras who posits that numbers are not dependent upon instantiations of them. We would do well to keep in mind that the Idealism associated with Pythagoras and Plato is not necessarily linked to the idealism associated with the ideal mate, the ideal baseball player, the ideal place to view a sunset, or even the ideal human. One who is an idealist in this latter sense is looking for the best fit given the set of really existing beings and places. One who is an Idealist in the former, Pythagorean and Platonic, sense argues for an ultimate reality beyond and underpinning the set of really existing beings and places.

Plato allies the human soul with the unchanging, immaterial Forms:

> Then the soul is more like the invisible than the body; and the body is like the visible. . . . Have we not also said that, when the soul employs the body in any inquiry, and makes use of sight or hearing, or any other sense — for inquiry with the body means inquiry of the sense — she is dragged away by it to the things which never remain the same, and wanders about blindly, and becomes confused and dizzy, like a drunken man, from dealing with things that are ever changing?. . . But when she investigates any question by herself, she goes away to the pure, and eternal, and immortal, and unchangeable, to which she is akin, and so she comes to be ever with it, as soon as she is by herself, and can be so; and then she rests from her wanderings and dwells with it unchangingly, for she is dealing with what is unchanging. And is not this state of the soul called wisdom?[25]

The trust that the soul shares characteristics with the enduring Forms and would, because of the shared characteristics, be most comfortable in their presence leads Socrates to proclaim that it would even be contradictory for the philosopher to fear death, since the philosopher, upon death, now is in the best possible place to live in harmony with the Forms. Of course, philosophy was not viewed by Socrates as the specialized, ivory tower discipline frequently associated with it. Anyone open to the pursuit of wisdom could become philosophical. This being the case, the open-minded *should not* fear death. If the open-minded acolytes surrounding Socrates as he grasped the hemlock in his final moments had such a view about death, Socrates wouldn't have had to console them with his arguments. Yet "we" now as "they" then are more consoled when death is put off, with staying alive, than with the stoic commandment "thou shalt not fear death." The cultural record we have just surveyed leads us to suppose that *once the Gilgameshian lesson that we will die is learned, humans look for permanence in the external* (laws, gods, institutions, Forms, etc.). Once the externals are established, human beings seek to live within that immortal structure and perhaps draw immortality from it.[26] This is what merging with the enduring is all about, and this is what we have really been examining since the first words of this book.

. . .

To fear death. We are back to our initial thoughts. We know we're going to die. We try all sorts of things to make our lives meaningful to ourselves and others. What makes us matter? What makes us worthy candidates for heaven or fame or any other variety of immortality? The Jew and Christian assert that we matter because we're made in the "image of God." For those who believe that deeds, not our substance, are most primary, the focus is on concrete accomplishments. Our accomplishments, intellectual and courageous, will live on, we hope. As they matter, we matter. The varieties of immortality may be inventions of self-justification, but even so, what wonderful inventions they are. Some may see them as failures to face reality, and others may see them as intimations of true reality. If they are mere chimeras, they help us sleep better. Yet if love, fame, creativity, spiritual aspirations, prolongevity, and merging with the enduring turn out to be attainable in the end, we gain life. Does the life we gain even roughly correspond to the concepts we now hold? It is impossible to know and so even the most learned among us must admit ignorance, even though the ignorance concerns those postulates so central to our self-worth.

APPENDIX: ORDERED LIST OF ARTWORK

CHAPTER ONE

Damien Hirst, *The Physical Impossibility of Death in the Mind of Someone Living*, 1991.

Francisco Goya, *Executions of the Third of May, 1808*

El Greco's *Burial of Count Orgaz*

Henry VIII by Hans Holbein

Plan for tomb of Julius II by Michelangelo, 1505.

Terra Cotta Army created under emperor Chin discovered in this century, but dating back over 2500 years.

Mausoleum at Halicarnassus

Nicolas Poussin, *I Too Once Dwelled in Arcady*

CHAPTER TWO

A Symposium Fresco from the Tomb of the Diver, c. 475BCE

J. B. Regnault, *Socrates Tears Alcibiades from the Embrace of Sensual Pleasure*, 1791

CHAPTER THREE

Jan Vermeer, *The Art of Painting*

Sandro Botticelli, *Adoration of the Magi*

Aegina Warrior (West Pediment: Parthenon)

Euripides, *Orestes Papyrus*

Leonardo Da Vinci, *Last Supper*

Marcel Duchamp, *Fountain*

Roettgen Pieta

CHAPTER FOUR

Marcel Duchamp, *Fountain*

Raphael, *Transfiguration*

Vermeer, *The Art of Painting*

Qutb Minar, India

Vendome Column, France

Portrait of a Couple, Pompeii

Chartres Cathedral, France

Raphael, *School of Athens*

Picasso, *Bull's Head*

Gino Severini, *Armored Train in Action*

Francisco Goya, *Third of May 1808*

Jacques Louis David, *Oath of the Horatii*

Edouard Manet, *The Execution of Emperor Maximilian*

Edouard Manet, *Olympia*

Titian, *Venus of Urbino*

Michelangelo, *Sistine Ceiling*

Khufu, *Great Pyramid*

CHAPTER SEVEN

Tomb of the Unknown Soldier

Ramses II, relief

Ramses II, in death

Kouros from Sounion

New York Kouros

Ptoon Kouros

Auxerre Kore

Peplos Kore

Parthenon

ENDNOTES

CHAPTER ONE

1. See Martin Heidegger, *Being In Time* (New York: Harper, 1962).

2. Benjamin R. Foster, translator and editor, *The Epic of Gilgamesh* (New York and London: W. W. Norton & Co., 2001), 47, 31–43.

3. This may be the allure of gladiator games, dog fights, and fatal car crashes. Death is experienced, but the observer is still living. Of course, the experienced death is not the death of the observer, and therefore, it is not the death that causes the existential distress noted by philosophers such as Martin Heidegger.

4. Sigmund Freud, "Thoughts for the Times on War and Death," tr. James Strachey, in *The Oxford Book of Death,* D. J. Enright, ed. (Oxford and New York : Oxford University Press, 1983), 153—154.

5. See Alan F. Segal *Life After Death: A History of the Afterlife in the Religions of the West* (New York: Doubleday, 2004), 86.

6. The plague seems to have aroused human consciousness of death for those who distracted themselves with other things. In our own day, terrorist attacks have similar effect even when the numbers killed are small in proportion to a population.

7. Giovanni Boccaccio, "The Decameron," Richard Aldington, trans., in *The Continental Edition of World Masterpieces, vol. 1,* Maynard Mack, ed. (New York: Norton 1966), 1012–1013.

8. We might understand why the human beings referred to by Boccaccio would do this, but I do not think any of us would praise their behavior. If one thinks of the progression of morals and mores from the Greeks to that late medieval period under present observation, we can note the steady attempts to take the basic kinship bonds of family and extend them. When Jesus taught the 'Our Father' prayer, he implies that we are all brothers and sisters under God (*Our* Father who art in heaven…). Before Jesus, Alexander the Great, perhaps with more self-serving ends, sought to intermarry the populations of Asia and Europe in hopes to widen the bonds of community. After Jesus, the Roman emperors would continue to promote the idea of

a universal family under the father of the country (*pater patriae*), a tradition adopted by the Church with the notion of the Pope (papa), or father of the universal Church on earth. But here with the Black Death, the kinship bonds proved to be less stable than previously thought.

9. Or, whether there is such a thing as a human soul that could exist separated from a body.

10. Natural theologians work from the real world back to God and infer things about God based upon his creation. They do not usually claim to have first-hand experience of God, although they in many cases claim to have knowledge of God.

11. One of the central concerns of cosmologists is cosmogony (how the universe began). Since the cosmologist was not around when, say, the big bang occurred, the cosmologist who believes in that hypothesis would not claim first-hand experience of how the universe began, although she may claim to have some knowledge of the event through the study of the present universe.

12. We do need to be careful here. That one has no first-hand experience of a lack of immortality does not entail that immortality awaits us. The point I make here is not about whether there *really* is immortality, it is that the experience of evidence can lead different people to believe that different concepts do or do not apply to reality.

13. We may experience others' fame for similar things and believe a qualitatively similar fame awaits us. Such was perhaps what Napoleon had in mind when he thought the enduring fame of Alexander the Great (for conquest) was to be his as well. Thanks to Peter N. Bonneau for this point.

14. John Donne, *Poems, by J. D. With elegies on the author's death* (Menston: Scholar Press, 1969).

15. Aubrey de Grey (with Michael Rae) *Ending aging : the rejuvenation breakthroughs that could reverse human aging in our lifetime* (New York : St. Martin's Press, 2007).

16. The carrying of a name, however, can prove to be a burden. Julian Lennon could not escape the comparisons to his father, John. Alexander the Great, on the other hand, benefited from his associations with his father Philip of Macedon, but was able to surpass his father's accomplishments.

17. Epicurus "Letter to Menoeceus," Russell M Geer, trans., in *Ancient Philosophy*, Forrest Baird and Walter Kaufmann, eds. (Upper Saddle River: Prentice Hall, 2003), 474. I should mention that Marcus Aurelius, the Stoic emperor, did not believe the future (or the past) could be "ours" since both future existence and the events of the past are beyond our control. It is unlikely that an immortalist would subscribe to Aurelius's brand of Stoicism since they seek to guarantee a future for themselves.

18. Propositions such as these are called 'analytic propositions,' because we can verify the truth of the relation between subject and predicate simply by analyzing, or looking into, the meaning of the concepts involved.

19. Corliss Lamont *The Illusion of Immortality* (New York: Continuum Publishing Company, 1990), 22.

20. Miguel de Unamuno puts the connection between death and immortality seeking in robust terms: "I do not want to die — no, I neither want to die nor do I want to want to die; I want to live for ever and ever and ever. I want this 'I' to live — this poor 'I' that I am and that I feel myself to be here and now, and therefore the

problem of the duration of my soul, of my own soul, tortures me." Miguel de Una-muno's *Tragic Sense of Life* (New York: Dover Publications, 1954), 60.

CHAPTER TWO

1. That is, he yearns to not-die and, so, he yearns to keep living. "To keep living" may take the form of (1) spiritual immortality, understood in this essay, as the soul's indefinite existence in another world or sphere, or (2) earthly immortality, understood in this book, as to continue recognizable life *in this world* with the personality intact. Gilgamesh seeks the latter (2).

2. Benjamin R. Foster, translator and editor, *The Epic of Gilgamesh* (New York and London: W. W. Norton & Co., 2001), 31–43, 47.

3. The obvious counterargument to this claim is the prevalence of "deadbeat dads," who drop out of the child's and former lover's life and extend neither money nor time to ensure the success of the offspring.

4. Benjamin R. Foster, translator and editor, *The Epic of Gilgamesh* (New York and London: W. W. Norton & Co., 2001), 5.

5. Goethe, *Faust: A Tragedy*, Martin Greenberg, trans. (New Haven: Yale, 1992), 98.

6. Goethe, *Faust: A Tragedy*, Martin Greenberg, trans. (New Haven: Yale, 1992), 98.

7. It is interesting to note that some would express endless love ("I'll love you forever") with increasing segments of time (—"Forever and a day") and even increasing (poetic) indefiniteness (" — Forever and ever").

8. *Matthew 22:29–30*

9. Thanks to Professor James Moody for this phrase. A serial monogamist goes from one exclusive relationship to the next in linear sequence.

10. See Derek Parfit's *Reasons and Persons* (Oxford: Clarendon Press, 1984), 165–85 for an example of a convincing account of our bias towards the future.

11. William Shakespeare, "Sonnet CXVI," in *Shakespeare's works* (New York: Funk & Wagnalls Co., 1899), 1025.

12. William Shakespeare, "Sonnet CXV," in *Shakespeare's works* (New York: Funk & Wagnalls Co., 1899), 1025.

13. Benjamin R. Foster, translator and editor, *The Epic of Gilgamesh* (New York and London: W. W. Norton & Co., 2001), 83.

14. Blaise Pascal, "Discourse on the Passion of Love," O. W. Wright, trans., in *The Harvard classics,* edited by Charles W. Eliot.(New York: P.F. Collier & Son, 1909–14), 22.

15. Robert G. Olson, *An Introduction to Existentialism* (New York: Dover Books, 1962), 18.

16. See Epictetus's *Encheiridion,* W.A. Oldfather, trans., in Baird and Kaufmann's (eds.) *Ancient Philosophy* (Upper Saddle River: Prentice Hall, 2003), 515–6: "What the will of nature is may be learned from a consideration of the points in which we do not differ from one another…Some other person's child or wife has died; no one but would say, 'Such is the fate of man.' Yet when a man's own child dies, immediately the cry is, 'Alas! Woe is me!' But we ought to remember how we feel when we hear of the same misfortune befalling others."

17. Tolstoy powerfully articulates this relation to the self: "He had been little Vanya, with a mamma and papa, afterwards with Katenka and with all the joys, griefs, and delights of childhood, boyhood, and youth. What did Caius know of the smell of that striped leather ball Vanya had been so fond of? Had Caius kissed his mother's hand like that? Could Caius preside at a session as he did? Caius really was mortal and it was right for him to die; but for me, little Vanya, Ivan Illych, with all my thoughts and emotions, it's altogether a different matter."

18. Luke 9:23–24. See also Mark 8:34 and Matthew 11:37.

19. John Hick, *Death and Eternal Life*, (San Francisco: Harper & Row, 1980), 66–7.

20. "The Laws of Manu" in Oliver. A. Johnson, ed., *Sources of World Civilization, Second Edition* (Upper Saddle River: Prentice Hall, 2000), 62–3.

21. Recall that Critias declared the gods to be an invention of a clever politician to secure orderly behavior even when authorities were not present to punish. The gods were always there to recognize transgressions.

22. Quoted in Mark T. Conrad's "God, Suicide, and the Meaning of Life," in *Woody Allen and Philosophy* (Peru, Illinois: Open Court, 2004), 21.

23. Leon Kass "The Wisdom of Repugnance: The Case against Human Cloning," in Christina Sommers and Fred Sommers' *Introductory Readings in Ethics* (Belmont: Wadsworth, 2004), 555. Originally in Leon R. Kass and James Q. Wilson *The Ethics of Cloning* (Washington, D.C.: American Enterprise Institute, 1998), 17–59.

24. *Hesiod's Theogony,* Norman 0. Brown, trans. (New York: Liberal Arts Press, 1953), 56–9, lines 116–153.

25. The purpose of Eros is to lead us to mate and bring forth new life. It is doubtful that Eros could be properly conceived independent of the Earth, which is that place where the mating and reproduction take place. Since the gods of the Greeks are immanent ("within nature") on Mt. Olympus, even the gods' erotic encounters would therefore presuppose the existence of the Earth. This could be different in other religions. For example, in Christianity, Eros would not require the existence of an earth. However, Christians would say that although it is logically possible for the goddess Eros to exist prior to and independent of an Earth, it is not in fact the case that there are any other gods besides God, understood as the Trinity.

26. This, it may be argued, would allow Socrates to maintain the position that he does not offer positive knowledge. He only purges others of false knowledge. The positive knowledge on love that he offers at the symposium comes from another source, Diotima, and not from Socrates.

27. Plato, *Symposium*, 211c3–7.

28. Recall Heraclitus who articulated that being itself is always changing. This view bothered Plato because one cannot be certain that one knows anything if the objects of study are not predictably stable.

29. Pythagoras is discussed at length in chapter seven of this book. He influentially argued that the essence of everything, including material things, was immaterial numbers. He is remembered as a formal monist, as contrasted with the material monists who believed that there was one principle to material things and that principle was an element of some sort (e.g., water).

30. *Symposium*, 211b5.

31. Anaximander is remembered for his notion of <apeiron>, or "the boundless," which helps in the explanation of the appearance of change in the material world even though, hitherto, philosophers thought that only four elements (water, earth, fire, air) underpinned the world. In a similar way, Plato believes that the Forms underpin the world. Anaximander is discussed in chapter 7.
32. Plato, *Phaedo*, 79b9–d5.

CHAPTER THREE

1. Yet, do not our children have to have children *ad infinitum* for this to bring us immortality through progeny? How confident could one really be in descendents' fortune and fertility if she pursued immortality through progeny? See, Robert Nozick, *Philosophical Explanations* (Boston: Harvard University Press), 1981.
2. *Symposium* 209c6–209e2.
3. Leo Strauss and Seth Benardete *Leo Strauss on Plato's Symposium* (Chicago: University of Chicago Press, 2001), 225.
4. Plato, *Republic*, Bk. V.
5. Daniel E Anderson, *The masks of Dionysos: a commentary on Plato's Symposium*, SUNY series in ancient Greek philosophy, (Albany, N.Y.: State University of New York Press, 1993), 79.
6. Plato, *Republic*, 428e7–429a1.
7. Plato, *Republic*, 428e7–429a1.
8. One of the five rivers in Hades.
9. Theocritus, in Roy T. Matthews's and F. DeWitt Platt's (eds.) *Readings in the Western humanities*, (Mountain View, Calif: Mayfield Pub., 2001), 89.
10. Shakespeare, "Sonnet LXXXI," in *Shakespeare's works* (New York: Funk & Wagnalls Co., 1899), 1020.
11. In our own time, some talk of former president Bill Clinton's concerns about his legacy and library as overpowering his desire to perform the kind of principled action that earns a good legacy. Fame can be accrued by conscious orchestration or as by-products of action. Fame is the goal and purpose in option one. It is a consequence and result in option two. I suspect most readers will consider the fame of option two to reflect better on the famous agent.
12. *Symposium* 208c2–e2.
13. Francis Bacon, "Of Fame," in *Essays and New Atlantis* (New York: Published for the Classics club by W.J. Black, 1942).
14. That is, we would be hard-pressed to deny the painting's independent value without committing the genetic fallacy. The genetic fallacy would be committed by erroneously basing the merits of the painting on the source of the painting. In truth, self-promoting individuals can produce great work.
15. Actually, the tragic poet Aeschylus (525–456 BCE) is more renowned for his drama did help defeat the Persians.
16. Plato, *The Apology*
17. Horace, "We All Must Die," Samuel Johnson, trans., in *Reading About the World*, Paul Brians, et. al., eds. (Harcourt Brace Custom, 1999).

18. Presumably, the music was written by Euripides himself. It is music from his tragedy *Orestes*. The actual papyrus, with the surviving notation, dates from a few centuries later.

19. This is the case, for example, with Da Vinci's famed masterpiece the *Battle of Anghiari*.

20. Otto Rank "Success and Fame," in the *The myth of the birth of the hero, and other writings,* Philip Freund, ed., (New York: Vintage Books, 1959), 219–221.

21. Marcus Aurelius, 529

22. The writer/character of Ecclesiastes is identified early in verse one as a Philosopher.

23. Ecclesiastes 1: 11, 16 *The Bible in Today's English Version*

24. Marcus Aurelius, 527.

25. Leo Strauss and Seth Benardete *Leo Strauss on Plato's Symposium* (Chicago: University of Chicago Press, 2001), 228.

26. *Phaedo* 79.

27. *Phaedo* 79d.

28. *Symposium* 211d5–212a3.

29. *Phaedo* 79d2.

30. *Symposium* 207d2–3.

31. William S. Cobb *The Symposium: and, The Phaedrus; Plato's erotic dialogues, SUNY series in ancient Greek philosophy* (Albany: State University of New York Press, 1993), 76.

32. *Symposium* 212b2.

33. *Symposium* 208b2–3

34. Anderson, 78.

35. *Apology* 40c3.

36. *Apology* 41b2–4.

37. I say "we can make" because there is no evidence within the Symposium itself that Socrates believes that fame needs personal immortality.

38. *Symposium* 200a6–b4.

39. *Phaedo* 66d6–e2.

40. *Symposium* 200d3–6.

41. Robert Nozick, "Death," in *The Experience of Philosophy*, Daniel Kolak and Raymond Martin, eds. (Belmont: Wadsworth, 1990), 367.

42. Francesco Petrarch, "On the Impossibility of Acquiring Fame During One's Lifetime, " in *The First Modern Scholar and Man of Letters: a selection from his correspondence with Boccaccio and other friends, designed to illustrate the beginnings of the Renaissance.* (London: GP Putnam's Sons, 1898), 409–414.

43. Francis Bacon, "Of Death," in *Essays and New Atlantis* (New York: Published for the Classics club by W.J. Black, 1942).

CHAPTER FOUR

1. "Artists Catch Head Lice for Show," BBC News, April 28, 2008, Entertainment section, http://news.bbc.co.uk/2/hi/entertainment/7370842.stm (Last Accessed: November 15, 2008).

2. That is, it has gotten as far as it could.

3. Fyodor Dostoevsky, "Notes from the Underground," David Magarshack, trans., in Gordon Marino's *Basic Writings of Existentialism* (New York: The Modern Library, 2004).

4. Otto Rank, "Life and Creation," in *The Myth of the Birth of the Hero and Other Writings*, Philip Freund, ed., (New York: Random House, 1964), 139–40

5. Alan Cowell, "More European Papers Print Cartoons of Muhammad, Fueling Dispute with Muslims," New York Times, Feb. 2, 2006, http://www.nytimes.com/2006/02/02/international/europe/02danish.html (Last Accessed: Feb 3, 2006).

6. A living religion is one that is still considered to be true. Christianity is a living religion, whereas the worship of Zeus is not. See William James's *The Will to Believe*

7. Emile Fackenheim, *God's Presence in History* (New York: Harper & Row, 1972), 84. Quoted in Lawrence S. Cunningham and John Kelsay *The Sacred Quest* (Upper Saddle River: Prentice Hall, 2002), 151.

8. E.M. Cioran, *The Trouble With Being Born* (New York: Viking Press, 1976), 73.

9. Andre Malraux, *The Creative Act*, in *The Psychology of Art: volume 2 of 3*, Stuart Gilbert, trans. (New York: Pantheon Books, 1949), 219.

10. Vincent Van Gogh, *Letter 506* (To his brother Theo), c.9 July 1888, R.G. Harrison, ed., 2001. http://www.vggallery.com/letters/619_V-T_506.pdf Last Accessed: November 18, 2008.

11. *Symposium*, 208e3–209b2.

12. For a philosophical schema of constrained choices in contemporary life, see Jason K. Swedene, *A Philosophy of Moral Dilemmas: Why We Should Not Feel Guilty About Things We Have Done* (Lewiston: Edwin Mellen Press, 2007).

13. Siddhartha Gautama left his family and ending up founding the Buddhist religion. Paul Gauguin left his family for the inspiration of Tahiti. He became a highly regarded and influential post-impressionist painter.

14. Josh Tyrangiel, "The Resurrection of Neil Young" *Time* Archive: Oct 3, 2005: http://www.time.com/time/acrchive/preview/0,10987,1109363,00.html, (Last accessed: 10/10/2005).

15. Cf. Paul Zelanski and Mary Pat Fisher, *The Art of Seeing* (Pearson, Upper Saddle River, 2007), 341.

16. See Woody Allen's one act play "Death Knocks" in *Without Feathers* (New York: Random House, 1975) for a humorous yet serious look at the many ways one might tell death to wait. On another point, the "I have a lot left to do" may be a reason many are unwilling to follow through with the utilitarian's claim that there are some times when the individual must sacrifice his life for others. The individual knows himself and tells himself what he will do and how serious he is about doing it. The individual, not knowing the others involved in the same way he knows himself, uses this insight into justify why his life is too valuable to sacrifice.

17. See Erich Heller's "Introduction" in *The Basic Kafka* (New York: Simon & Schuster, 1979), ix–xxvii.

18. For examples of creative products recollected but no longer in existence, consider such monumental works as Phidias's Athena, Mausolos's tomb, Old St. Peter's, and the Abbey Church at Cluny.

19. Bertrand Russell, "A Free Man's Worship," in *Why I am not a Christian, and other essays on religion and related subjects* (New York: Simon and Schuster, 1957).

CHAPTER FIVE

1. The Socratic Method is characterized by mixing inquiry with dialogue to obtain reliable clarification and definition.

2. No written works from Socrates have come down to us, and it is generally agreed that he did not write any thing of philosophical significance.

3. We need not sort out what Socrates *actually thought* (i.e., whether his convictions were closer to the *Apology* or *Phaedo*) in the days leading up to his death to evaluate his *arguments* about the soul and personal immortality.

4. Plato, *Phaedo*, 64a4.

5. Plato (*Phaedo*, 66d6–e3) writes: "Verily we have learned that if we are to have any pure knowledge at all, we must be freed from the body; the soul by herself must behold things as they are." The senses often trick us into thinking we know something and so, for Socrates, we would be all the better for jettisoning them.

6. The ka had to find its way back to its correct body. To this purpose art was very realistic with slight modifications of posture tolerable.

7. The pyramid design, each time it's used, echoes the Egyptians' use of it. See for example, IM Pei's *Louvre Pyramid* in Paris, France and the *Transamerica Building* in San Francisco, California (USA).

8. *Exodus 26–27*

9. "The Book of Job," in *Sources of World Civilization, v. I, To 1500*, Oliver A. Johnson, ed., (Upper Saddle River, NJ: Prentice Hall, 2000), 48.

10. *Genesis 12*.

11. Even in the Mesopotamian *Gilgamesh*, Utnapishtim equates sleep and death, challenging Gilgamesh to overcome days of not sleeping to show himself ready to overcome death.

12. See *Matthew 19:30*.

13. See, again, Miguel de Unamuno's moving plea: "I do not want to die—no, I neither want to die nor do I want to want to die; I want to live for ever and ever and ever. I want this 'I' to live—this poor 'I' that I am and that I feel myself to be here and now, and therefore the problem of the duration of my soul, of my own soul, tortures me." Miguel de Unamuno's *Tragic Sense of Life* (New York: Dover Publications, 1954), 60.

14. *Ecclesiastes* 3: 21-22. See also *Ecclesiastes* 6:12 and *Ecclesiastes* 10:14

15. *Ecclesiastes* 4:1-3

16. *Ecclesiastes* 9:3-5. Is a living victim of continuous physical and emotional abuse better off than a dead Lorenzo the Magnificent simply because the victim is alive *now,* rather than Lorenzo who seems to have had a pretty good life and had a similarly experienced *now* that spanned the years prior to the victim presently living? Everyone's *now* will be past. Should those who possess a *now* be regarded as luckier or better off than those who had a *now* in the past?

17. *Psalms* 88:4-7.

18. *Wisdom* 2: 1-4.

19. *John 18:36.*

20. Fyodor Dostoyevsky examines one consequence of a heavenly kingdom in his *Brothers Karamazov:* Had Jesus proclaimed his kingdom to be of this world, he could have offered guidance applicable to this life. In a word, if the goal is an earthly kingdom, then the means to get there could be set out in terms of concrete earthly acts to achieve that kingdom. With a heavenly kingdom, however, humans do not have the means set out for them. See Fyodor Dostoevsky, *Brothers Karamazov*, in Marino's *Basic Writings of Existentialism,* David Magarshack, trans., in Gordon Marino's *Basic Writings of Existentialism* (New York: The Modern Library, 2004), 244–245.

21. *Isaiah 14.*

22. See *Isaiah 7:14, Isaiah 9:5* and *Isaiah 53:1–12.*

23. *Matthew 22: 21.*

24. *Matthew 6: 10.*

25. *2 Peter 3: 10.*

26. *Matthew 25: 41–46.*

27. *1 Corinthians 15: 56.*

28. *1 Corinthians 15: 21–22.*

29. *1 Corinthians 15: 36–44.* See John Hick, *Death and Eternal Life,* (San Francisco: Harper & Row, 1980), 185.

30. Late baroque artists (c. late 1600s) had similar difficulty portraying divine love, so they tended to place cupids in divine places.

31. John Hick, *Death and Eternal Life,* (San Francisco: Harper & Row, 1980), 177.

32. See, for example, *Revelation* 4 through 21 in which paradise is service to God rather than an extension of earthly activities. This theme is emphasized in *Luke* 20: 28—35 where, as was noted in our discussion of love, Jesus instructs his followers that the extension of marriage into the afterlife does not occur in heaven.

33. This is the holy book of Islam revealed, word for word, to Muhammad beginning in 610 CE. *Koran* and *Qu'ran* are both acceptable spellings.

34. *Matthew 25:31–45.*

35. Charity may be in this case equated with the morally supererogatory, which is morally good action that comes with a high recommendation. Requirements, on the other hand, are obligatory. Almsgiving is not recommended, but required.

36. *Surah 9:103, Surah 73:20.*

37. *Surah 56: 5 Anthology of World Scriptures*, Robert E. Van Voorst, ed. (Belmont, CA: Wadsworth Pub., 2006).

38. *Surah 69: 20 Anthology of World Scriptures*, Robert E. Van Voorst, ed. (Belmont, CA: Wadsworth Pub., 2006).

39. *Surah 76: 10, 15. Anthology of World Scriptures*, Robert E. Van Voorst, ed. (Belmont, CA: Wadsworth Pub., 2006).

40. *Surah 56: 15 Anthology of World Scriptures*, Robert E. Van Voorst, ed. (Belmont, CA: Wadsworth Pub., 2006).

41. *Surah 56: 20 Anthology of World Scriptures*, Robert E. Van Voorst, ed. (Belmont, CA: Wadsworth Pub., 2006).

42. 'houris'— "dark-eyed, beautiful women"

43. *Surah 56: 15, 35* and Hadith, 320 from *Anthology of World Scriptures*, Robert E. Van Voorst, ed. (Belmont, CA: Wadsworth Pub., 2006).

44. Indeed, *Jannah* (Arabic for 'heaven') means "garden."

45. *Surah* 47:15, Robert E. Van Voorst, ed. (Belmont, CA: Wadsworth Pub., 2006).

46. *Surah* 56:34-37, Robert E. Van Voorst, ed. (Belmont, CA: Wadsworth Pub., 2006).

47. *Surah* 69:30, Robert E. Van Voorst, ed. (Belmont, CA: Wadsworth Pub., 2006).

48. *Surah* 69: 25-35, Robert E. Van Voorst, ed. (Belmont, CA: Wadsworth Pub., 2006).

49. Surah 77: 21-29, Robert E. Van Voorst, ed. (Belmont, CA: Wadsworth Pub., 2006).

50. Surah 77: 29, Robert E. Van Voorst, ed. (Belmont, CA: Wadsworth Pub., 2006).

51. Surah 69: 35, Robert E. Van Voorst, ed. (Belmont, CA: Wadsworth Pub., 2006).

52. Surah 77: 30-35, Robert E. Van Voorst, ed. (Belmont, CA: Wadsworth Pub., 2006).

53. Surah 56: 24, Robert E. Van Voorst, ed. (Belmont, CA: Wadsworth Pub., 2006).

54. Surah 77: 35, Robert E. Van Voorst, ed. (Belmont, CA: Wadsworth Pub., 2006).

55. This section has been much improved by conversations with and writings of Fulbright Scholar Rachida El Diwani, who visited LSSU in the fall of 2005.

56. "The Hymns of the Rig Veda," Ralph T. H. Griffith, trans., in *The Human Record: Sources of Global History* Alfred J. Andrea and James H Overfield, eds. (Boston and New York: Houghton Mifflin, 1998), 27.

57. *The Bible of the World,* Robert O. Bellou, ed. (New York: Viking, 1939), 250–251, quoted in Jiu-Hwi Upshur, et. al, *World History* (Belmont: Wadsworth, 2002), 57.

58. See *The Human Record: Sources of Global History,* Alfred J. Andrea and James H Overfield, eds. (Boston and New York: Houghton Mifflin, 1998), 70.

59. Being "lost" is not equivalent to being "annihilated." An entity "lost" may nevertheless maintain its existence, as when someone loses their car keys. Of course, what is lost may be "gone," as when someone "loses" his parent to death.

60. See *The Human Record: Sources of Global History,* Alfred J. Andrea and James H Overfield, eds. (Boston and New York: Houghton Mifflin, 1998), 76–7.

61. Buddhist cultures influenced by this thought would obviously place little importance, if any, on living on through one's offspring and the intimate fame made possible by having descendants.

62. James Rachels, *The Elements of Moral Philosophy* (New York: Random House, 1986).

63. John Hick "Toward a Philosophy of Religious Pluralism," *Neue Zeitschrift fur Systematische Theologie und Religionphilosophie,* 22, 1980, 131–149.

CHAPTER SIX

1. Who one was in the Middle Ages was inseparable from the work one did. One *was* a king or a peasant, and so on. Despite the Renaissance influence that we might choose a non-traditional life and transform ourselves in the process, the Reformation idea of being "born again," and the Baroque emphasis on transformation, we now seem to be getting back to the idea that we are what we do.

2. See The President's Commission for the Study of Ethical Problems in Medicine and Biomedical and Behavioral Research, *Defining Death: A Report on the Medical, Legal, and Ethical Issues in the Determination of Death* (Washington, D.C.: US Government Printing Office, 1981), 12–43.

3. Leonard Hayflick, "Perspectives on Human Longevity," in *Extending the human life span: social policy and social ethics,* Bernice Levin Neugarten and Robert James Havighurst, eds. (Chicago: University of Chicago, 1977).

4. William R. Clark, *A Means to an End: The Biological Basis of Aging and Death* (New York and Oxford: Oxford University Press, 1999), 15.

5. It should be noted that Abraham, the patriarch of three faiths, is said to have died at "the ripe old age" of 175. We would expect Abraham, given his importance, to have lived longer. This, of course, challenges the exaltation-of-ancestors theory. Yet, on the other hand, this new standard for longevity, while quite a bit less than for Methuselah, is said to be the result of the wickedness of mankind around Noah's time (Methuselah's grandson) leading to God shortening the lifespan to 120 (see *Genesis 6:3*). In this revised lifespan frame, Abraham has outlived the amended human lifespan by more than forty percent.

6. *Genesis 5:22–24*

7. *Genesis 5:25–27*

8. Robert A. Heinlein, *Methuselah's Children* (New York: The New American Library, 1958).

9. Henry J. Aaron and William B. Schwartz, "Coping with Methuselah: Public Policy Implications of a Lengthening Human Life Span," *The Brookings Review*, Fall 2003, Vol. 21, No. 4, 36–39.

10. Even the belief that fame does not provide true, objective immortality must be regarded as uncertain. Perhaps people on earth will remember the famous and pass down the memory to others who remember. Perhaps the universe will not come to an end precluding this transference of memory. If earthly memory turns out to be unsustainable, there may yet be a heaven in which memories are maintained, restored, and given new information. In any case, whether memory survives on earth or in a paradise, one would have to be immortal to verify that memory survived intact.

11. The difference between our value being hinged to the species and our value being hinged to God is precisely that, in the case of species valuation, the individual is expendable: it does not matter if the individual is lost as long as the species prospers. With God, the individual may be a portion of the divine (Hinduism) or "good" and valuable in the eyes of God (Judaism, Christianity, Islam). If value is connected to God, the individual is not expendable.

12. Ludwig Wittgenstein, *Tractatus logico-philosophicus* (London: Routledge & Paul, 1961), 6.4312.

13. This is what tortures Garcin so much in Jean Paul Sartre's *No exit.* He judges himself a coward and cannot refrain from doing so given an eternity of time to examine his actions from his time on earth. See Jean-Paul Sartre, *No exit and three other plays* (New York: Vintage International, 1989).

14. I invite the reader to think of examples of fleeting events that happen later in life that are celebrated by our culture. One might be the event of having a first grandchild. Unlike the other examples in the list, though, having a first grandchild is a fleeting event that *happens* to the grandparent, rather than an activity that the grandparent *takes part* in like a first date.

15. Luke 9:24

16. St. Benedict, *The rule of Saint Benedict*, Francis Aidan Gasquet, trans. (New York: Cooper Square Publishers, 1966).

17. Pascal, "Pensees (Thoughts)" Baird and Kaufmann, 111.

18. James Merrill, "The Immortal Husband," in James Merrill's *Collected Novels and Plays*, J.D. McClatchy and Steven Yenser (eds.) (New York: Alfred A. Knopf, 2002), 541–543.

19. Alfred L. Tennyson "Tithonus," *Poems and plays* (London: Oxford University Press, 1967).

20. William R. Clark, *A means to an end: the biological basis of aging and death* (New York: Oxford University Press, 1999), 4.

21. The ship of Theseus is often invoked as a problem of identity. If you replace the parts of a ship one by one, at what point does the ship become a different ship? Considering the body as a ship of Theseus: I suppose that if one could replace all the parts of one's body, the end-result body would be an altogether new body. But unless the part-replacement were perpetual, even the new bodies would age. If the part-replacement were perpetual and thus resulted in continuous new bodies, this would hardly be the biological immortality we think of as normally sought or optimally worth seeking: ceaseless receipt of the most invasive health care.

22. Kant's most accessible moral treatise is his classic *Groundwork for the Metaphysics of Morals,* H. J. Paton, ed. *Groundwork of the metaphysic of moral* (New York: Harper & Row, 1964). In Book II, he explores the notion of duty. Duty, Kant concludes is what ought to be done regardless of what one wants to do. Plato's *Crito* endorses a similar notion of duty, with Socrates telling Crito that duty sometimes requires that we act against our inclinations.

23. John Hardwig, "Is There a Duty to Die?," in *Ethical issues in modern medicine: contemporary readings in bioethics*, Bonnie Steinbock, John Arras, and Alex John London, eds. (Boston: McGraw-Hill, 2009), 511–520.

24. I assume that some immortals are nevertheless susceptible to death by accident or natural calamity.

25. Karel Capek, "The Makropulos Secret" in *Toward the Radical Center: A Karel Capek Reader*, Peter Kussi, (New Jersey: Catbird Press, 1990), 162.

26. Karel Capek, "The Makropulos Secret" in *Toward the Radical Center: A Karel Capek Reader*, Peter Kussi ed. (New Jersey: Catbird Press, 1990), 170–171.

27. See David M. Friedman, *The Immortalists: Charles Lindbergh, Dr. Alexis Carrel, and Their Daring Quest to Live Forever* (New York: Harper Collins Publishers, 2007).

28. If this is true, then would a permanent life in heaven also lose its meaning too?

29. Karel Capek, "The Makropulos Secret" in *Toward the Radical Center: A Karel Capek Reader*, Peter Kussi, ed. (New Jersey: Catbird Press, 1990), 174.

30. David E. Bloom, David Canning, and Jaypee Sevilla *Demographic Divided: New Perspective on Economic Consequences of Population Change* (New York: The Rand Corporation, 2003).

CHAPTER SEVEN

1. Ric Burns, Marilyn Ness, David Ogden Stiers, and Li-Shin Yu.. *Ansel Adams a documentary film.* (Alexandria, VA: PBS DVD Video, 2002).

2. The prolongevitor depends on the Earth to comply as much as the lover of God needs Him to comply.

3. Plato, *Symposium* 191c–d5.

4. *John 3:16*

5. Blaise Pascal, *Pensees*, Quoted in the *Oxford Book of Death*, D.J. Enright, ed. (Oxford and New York: Oxford University Press, 1983), 156–7.

6. It seems that the fame of "must-see" movies and fictional characters bestow a similar identity to the group of "rememberers" without being thought of as granting continued life to the famous, for the reason that the famous never existed.

7. Although maybe its haziness allows for a certain degree of romanticizing, similar to what the haziness of nostalgia can do for events of the past.

8. Miguel de Unamuno, *The Tragic Sense of Life* (New York: Dover Publications, 1954), 65–87.

9. Miguel de Unamuno, "San Manuel Bueno, Martyr" in *Abel Sanchez and Other Stories*, Anthony Kerrigan, trans. (Washington, D.C.: Regnery Publishing Co., 1956).

10. *John 9:4*

11. See *Matthew 5*

12. Following Pascal, Miguel de Unamuno puts it well: "It is just as gratuitous to exist at all as to go on existing forever." See his *The Tragic Sense of Life* (New York: Dover Publications, 1954), 53.

13. *Exodus 20*

14. Thomas Jefferson, *Declaration of Independence*, 1776.

15. Can the anonymous have a reputation?

16. "Soldier in Tomb of Unknowns May Actually Be Known," *CNN.com*, January 20 1998, http://www.cnn.com/ALLPOLITICS/1998/01/20/unknown.soldier/, (Last accessed: 11/18/2008).

17. The term *<apeiron>* has no precise and sufficient translation. Following established precedent, I present the term in its untranslated form.

18. Anaximander, Fragment, in *Philosophic classics*, Forrest E. Baird and Walter Arnold Kaufmann, eds. (Upper Saddle River, N.J.: Prentice Hall, 2003), 10. Fragment taken from St. Augustine's *City of God*, VIII, 2; K146.

19. Ludwig Feuerbach, *Thoughts on Death and Immortality*. James A. Massey, ed. (Berkeley, Los Angeles, and London: University of California Press, 1980), 137.

20. Victor Davis Hanson *Carnage and Culture* (Doubleday: NY, 2001).

21. Victor Davis Hanson *Carnage and Culture* (Doubleday: NY, 2001).

22. Cicero, "The Dream of Scipio" from *De republica*, HA Rice, trans. Reprinted in *Continental Masterpieces*, Maynard Mack (general editor) (New York: WW Norton & Co., 1966), 607.

23. Quoted in *Philosophic classics*, Forrest E. Baird and Walter Arnold Kaufmann, eds. (Upper Saddle River, N.J.: Prentice Hall, 2003), from Sextus Empiricus, translated as *Against the Physicists* 1.54, by R. C. Bury in *Sextus Empiricus*, 3.31 sq. (London: W. Heinemann, 1936).

24. Aristotle, *Politics* 1253a3–4 and 1253a31–32.

25. Plato, *Phaedo* 79

26. Plato, in fact, believed that the soul is "akin" to the forms and the deceased philosopher dwells in contemplation of them. Christians would express this as: (1) God is the source and sustainer of all life, and so (2) the souls of the deceased who dwell in heaven get their life from God.

BIBLIOGRAPHY

"Artists Catch Head Lice for Show," BBC News, April 28, 2008, Entertainment section, http://news.bbc.co.uk/2/hi/entertainment/7370842.stm/, Last Accessed: 11/15/2008.

"Soldier in Tomb of Unknowns May Actually Be Known," *CNN.com*, January 20 1998, http://www.cnn.com/ALLPOLITICS/1998/01/20/unknown.soldier/, Last accessed: 11/18/2008.

"The Book of Job," In *Sources of World Civilization, v. I, To 1500*, edited by Oliver A. Johnson. Upper Saddle River, NJ: Prentice Hall, 2000.

"The Hymns of the Rig Veda," translated by Ralph T. H. Griffith, In *The Human Record: Sources of Global History*, edited by Alfred J. Andrea and James H Overfield. Boston and New York: Houghton Mifflin, 1998.

"The Laws of Manu" In *Sources of World Civilization, Second Edition*. edited by Oliver. A. Johnson. Upper Saddle River: Prentice Hall, 2000.

Aaron, Henry J., and William B. Schwartz. "Coping with Methuselah: Public Policy Implications of a Lengthening Human Life Span," *The Brookings Review*, Fall 2003, Vol. 21, No. 4, 36–39.

Cowell, Alan. "More European Papers Print Cartoons of Muhammad, Fueling Dispute with Muslims," New York Times, Feb. 2, 2006, http://www.nytimes.com/2006/02/02/international/europe/02danish.html, Last Accessed: Feb 3, 2006.

Allen, Woody. "Death Knocks" in *Without Feathers*. New York: Random House, 1975.

Anaximander. "Fragment", In *Philosophic classics, vol. 1: Ancient Philosophy*, edited by Forrest E. Baird and Walter Arnold Kaufmann. Upper Saddle River, N.J.: Prentice Hall, 2003, 10. Fragment taken from St. Augustine's *City of God*, VIII, 2; K146.

Anderson, Daniel E. *The masks of Dionysos: a commentary on Plato's Symposium*. Albany, N.Y.: State University of New York Press, 1993.

Andre Malraux. *The Creative Act*, In *The Psychology of Art: volume 2 of 3*, translated by Stuart Gilbert. New York: Pantheon Books, 1949.

Aristotle. *Politics,* In *The basic works of Aristotle,* edited by Richard Peter McKeon. New York: Modern Library, 2001.

Aurelius, Marcus. "Meditations," In *Ancient Philosophy,* Forrest Baird and Walter Kaufmann, eds. Upper Saddle River: Prentice Hall, 2003.

Bacon, Francis. "Of Death," In *Essays and New Atlantis.* New York: Published for the Classics club by W.J. Black, 1942.

Bloom, David E., David Canning, and Jaypee Sevilla. *Demographic Divided: New Perspective on Economic Consequences of Population Change.* New York: The Rand Corporation, 2003.

Boccaccio, Giovanni. "The Decameron," Richard Aldington, trans., in *The Continental Edition of World Masterpieces, vol. 1,* Maynard Mack, ed. New York: Norton, 1966.

Hesiod. *Hesiod's Theogony,* translated by Norman 0. Brown. New York: Liberal Arts Press, 1953.

Burns, Ric, Marilyn Ness, David Ogden Stiers, and Li-Shin Yu. *Ansel Adams a documentary film.* Alexandria, VA: PBS DVD Video, 2002.

Capek,Karel. "The Makropulos Secret." in *Toward the Radical Center: A Karel Capek Reader,* Peter Kussi, ed. New Jersey: Catbird Press, 1990, 162.

Catholic Biblical Association of America, and Confraternity of Christian Doctrine. *Genesis.* In *The new American Bible.* New York: P.J. Kenedy, 1970.

Catholic Biblical Association of America, and Confraternity of Christian Doctrine. *Matthew.* In *The new American Bible.* New York: P.J. Kenedy, 1970.

Catholic Biblical Association of America, and Confraternity of Christian Doctrine. *Psalms.* In *The new American Bible.* New York: P.J. Kenedy, 1970.

Catholic Biblical Association of America, and Confraternity of Christian Doctrine. *Wisdom.* In *The new American Bible.* New York: P.J. Kenedy, 1970.

Catholic Biblical Association of America, and Confraternity of Christian Doctrine. *Ecclesiastes.* In *The new American Bible.* New York: P.J. Kenedy, 1970.

Catholic Biblical Association of America, and Confraternity of Christian Doctrine. *John.* In *The new American Bible.* New York: P.J. Kenedy, 1970.

Catholic Biblical Association of America, and Confraternity of Christian Doctrine. *Isaiah.* In *The new American Bible.* New York: P.J. Kenedy, 1970.

Catholic Biblical Association of America, and Confraternity of Christian Doctrine. *2 Peter.* In *The new American Bible.* New York: P.J. Kenedy, 1970.

Catholic Biblical Association of America, and Confraternity of Christian Doctrine. *1 Corinthians.* In *The new American Bible.* New York: P.J. Kenedy, 1970.

Catholic Biblical Association of America, and Confraternity of Christian Doctrine. *Revelation.* In *The new American Bible.* New York: P.J. Kenedy, 1970.

Catholic Biblical Association of America, and Confraternity of Christian Doctrine. *Luke.* In *The new American Bible.* New York: P.J. Kenedy, 1970.

Cicero. "The Dream of Scipio" from *De republica,* HA Rice, trans. Reprinted in *Continental Masterpieces,* Maynard Mack, ed. New York: WW Norton & Co., 1966, 607.

Cioran, E.M. *The Trouble With Being Born.* New York: Viking Press, 1976.

Clark, William R. *A means to an end: the biological basis of aging and death.* New York: Oxford University Press, 1999.

Clark, William R. *A Means to an End: The Biological Basis of Aging and Death.* New York and Oxford: Oxford University Press, 1999.

Cobb, William S. *The Symposium and The Phaedrus; Plato's erotic dialogues, SUNY series in ancient Greek philosophy.* Albany: State University of New York Press, 1993.

Conard, Mark T. and Aeon J. Skoble. eds. *Woody Allen and philosophy: you mean my whole fallacy is wrong?, Popular culture and philosophy,* v. 8. Chicago: Open Court, 2004.

De Grey, Aubrey, with Michael Rae, *Ending aging: the rejuvenation breakthroughs that could reverse human aging in our lifetime.* New York : St. Martin's Press, 2007.

Donne, John. *Poems, by J. D. With elegies on the author's death.* Menston: Scholar Press, 1969.

Dostoevsky, Fyodor *Brothers Karamazov,* translated by David Magarshack, In *Basic Writings of Existentialism,* edited by Gordon Marino. New York: The Modern Library, 2004.

Fackenheim, Emile. *God's Presence in History.* New York: Harper & Row, 1972.

Cunningham Lawrence S., and John Kelsay. *The Sacred Quest.* Upper Saddle River: Prentice Hall, 2002, 151.

Epictetus. *Encheiridion,* translated by W.A. Oldfather, In *Ancient Philosophy,* edited by Forrest Baird and Walter Kaufmann. Upper Saddle River: Prentice Hall, 2003.

Epicurus. "Letter to Menoeceus," translated by Russell M. Geer, In *Ancient Philosophy,* edited by Forrest Baird and Walter Kaufmann. Upper Saddle River: Prentice Hall, 2003.

Feuerbach, Ludwig. *Thoughts on Death and Immortality,* edited by James A. Massey. Berkeley, Los Angeles, and London: University of California Press, 1980.

Foster, Benjamin R., translator and editor, *The Epic of Gilgamesh.* New York and London: W. W. Norton & Co., 2001.

Bacon, Francis. "Of Fame," In *Essays and New Atlantis.* New York: Published for the Classics club by W.J. Black, 1942.

Freud, Sigmund. "Thoughts for the Times on War and Death," translated by James Strachey, In *The Oxford Book of Death,* edited by D. J. Enright. Oxford and New York: Oxford University Press, 1983.

Friedman, David M. *The Immortalists: Charles Lindbergh, Dr. Alexis Carrel, and Their Daring Quest to Live Forever.* New York: Harper Collins Publishers, 2007.

Fyodor Dostoevsky, "Notes from the Underground", translated by David Magarshack, In *Basic Writings of Existentialism,* edited by Gordon Marino,. New York: The Modern Library, 2004.

Goethe, Johann Wolfgang von, *Faust, a tragedy. Part 1,* translated by Martin Greenberg. New Haven: Yale University Press, 1992.

Hanson, Victor Davis. *Carnage and Culture.* Doubleday: NY, 2001.

Hardwig, John. "Is There a Duty to Die?" In *Ethical Issues in Modern Medicine: Contemporary Readings in Bioethics,* edited by Bonnie Steinbock, John Arras, and Alex John London. Boston: McGraw-Hill, 2009.

Heidegger, Martin. *Being in Time.* New York: Harper, 1962.

Heinlein, Robert A. *Methuselah's Children.* New York: The New American Library, 1958.

Heller, Erich. "Introduction," In *The Basic Kafka.* New York: Simon & Schuster, 1979.

Hick, John. *Death and Eternal Life.* San Francisco: Harper & Row, 1980.

Horace. "We All Must Die," translated by Samuel Johnson, In *Reading About the World,* edited by Paul Brians, et. al. Harcourt Brace Custom, 1999.

James, William. *The will to believe, and other essays in popular philosophy, and Human immortality*. New York: Dover Publications, 1960.

Jefferson, Thomas. The *Declaration of Independence*, 1776, usahistory.com, http://www.ushistory.org/Declaration/document/index.htm, Last accessed: 11/20/2008.

Hick, John. "Toward a Philosophy of Religious Pluralism," *Neue Zeitschrift fur Systematische Theologie und Religionphilosophie*, 22, 1980, 131–149.

Kant, Immanuel. *Groundwork for the metaphysics of morals*. H. J. Paton, ed. New York: Harper & Row, 1964.

Kass, Leon R. "The Wisdom of Repugnance: The Case against Human Cloning," In Christina Sommers and Fred Sommers' *Introductory Readings in Ethics*. Belmont: Wadsworth, 2004.

Kass, Leon R., and James Q. Wilson. *The Ethics of Cloning*. Washington, D.C.: American Enterprise Institute, 1998.

Lamont, Corliss. *The Illusion of Immortality*. New York: Continuum Publishing Company, 1990.

Leonard Hayflick, "Perspectives on Human Longevity," In *Extending the human life span: social policy and social ethics,* edited by Bernice Levin Neugarten and Robert James Havighurst. Chicago: University of Chicago, 1977.

Merrill, James. *Collected Novels and Plays*, edited by J.D. McClatchy and Steven Yenser. New York: Alfred A. Knopf, 2002.

Nozick, Robert. "Death," In *The Experience of Philosophy*, edited by Daniel Kolak and Raymond Martin. Belmont: Wadsworth, 1990.

Nozick, Robert. *Philosophical Explanations*. Boston: Harvard University Press, 1981.

Olson, Robert G. *An Introduction to Existentialism.* .New York: Dover Books,

Parfit, Derek. *Reasons and Persons*. Oxford: Clarendon Press, 1984.

Pascal, Blaise. in *Philosophic classics, vol. 3: Modern Philosophy.*

Pascal, Blaise. "Pensees," Quoted in the *Oxford Book of Death*, edited by D.J. Enright. Oxford and New York: Oxford University Press, 1983, 156–7.

Pascal, Blaise. "Discourse on the Passion of Love," translated by O. W. Wright, In *The Harvard classics,* edited by Charles W. Eliot. New York: P.F. Collier & Son, 1909–14.

Petrarch, Francesco. "On the Impossibility of Acquiring Fame During One's Lifetime," In *The First Modern Scholar and Man of Letters: a selection from his correspondence with Boccaccio and other friends, designed to illustrate the beginnings of the Renaissance*. London: GP Putnam's Sons, 1898.

Plato. *Apology,* In *Ancient Philosophy,* edited by Forrest Baird and Walter Kaufmann, eds. Upper Saddle River: Prentice Hall, 2003.

Plato. *Crito,* In *Ancient Philosophy,* edited by Forrest Baird and Walter Kaufmann, eds. Upper Saddle River: Prentice Hall, 2003.

Plato. *Phaedo,* In *Ancient Philosophy,* edited by Forrest Baird and Walter Kaufmann, eds. Upper Saddle River: Prentice Hall, 2003.

Plato. *Republic,* In *Ancient Philosophy,* edited by Forrest Baird and Walter Kaufmann, eds. Upper Saddle River: Prentice Hall, 2003.

Plato. *Symposium,* In *Ancient Philosophy,* edited by Forrest Baird and Walter Kaufmann, eds. Upper Saddle River: Prentice Hall, 2003.

Rachels, James. *The Elements of Moral Philosophy*. New York: Random House, 1986.

Rank, Otto. "Life and Creation," In *The Myth of the Birth of the Hero and Other Writings*, edited by Philip Freund. New York: Random House, 1964.

Rank, Otto. "Success and Fame," In *The Myth of the Birth of the Hero and Other Writings*, edited by Philip Freund. New York: Random House, 1964.

Russell Bertrand. "A Free Man's Worship," In *Why I am not a Christian, and other essays on religion and related subjects*. New York: Simon and Schuster, 1957.

Sartre, Jean-Paul. *No exit and three other plays*. New York: Vintage International, 1981.

Segal, Alan F. *Life After Death: A History of the Afterlife in the Religions of the West*. New York: Doubleday, 2004.

Shakespeare, William. "Sonnet CXV," In *Shakespeare's works*. New York: Funk & Wagnalls Co., 1899, 1025.

Shakespeare, William "Sonnet CXVI," In *Shakespeare's works*. New York: Funk & Wagnalls Co., 1899, 1025.

Shakespeare, William, "Sonnet LXXXI," In *Shakespeare's works*. New York: Funk & Wagnalls Co., 1899, 1020.

St. Benedict. *The rule of Saint Benedict*, translated by Francis Aidan Gasquet. New York: Cooper Square Publishers, 1966.

Strauss, Leo and Seth Benardete. *Leo Strauss on Plato's 'Symposium'*. Chicago: University of Chicago Press, 2001.

Swedene, Jason K. *A Philosophy of Moral Dilemmas: Why We Should Not Feel Guilty About Things We Have Done*. Lewiston: Edwin Mellen Press, 2007.

Tennyson, Alfred L. "Tithonus," In *Poems and plays*. London: Oxford University Press, 1967.

The Bible of the World, edited by Robert O. Bellou, ed. New York: Viking, 1939.

The Human Record: Sources of Global History, edited by Alfred J. Andrea and James H. Overfield. Boston and New York: Houghton Mifflin, 1998.

The President's Commission for the Study of Ethical Problems in Medicine and Biomedical and Behavioral Research, *Defining Death: A Report on the Medical, Legal, and Ethical Issues in the Determination of Death*. Washington, D.C.: US Government Printing Office, 1981, 12–43.

Theocritus. *Readings in the Western humanities*, edited by Roy T. Matthews and F. DeWitt Platt. Mountain View, Calif: Mayfield Pub., 2001.

Tyrangiel, Josh. "The Resurrection of Neil Young" *Time* Archive: Oct 3, 2005: http://www.time.com/time/acrchive/preview//0,10987,1109363,00.html, Last accessed: 10/10/2005.

Unamuno y Jugo, Miguel de. "San Manuel Bueno, Martyr, " translated by Anthony Kerrigan, In *Abel Sanchez and Other Stories*. Washington, D.C.: Regnery Publishing Co., 1956.

Unamuno y Jugo, Miguel de. *The Tragic Sense of Life*. New York: Dover Publications, 1954.

Van Gogh, Vincent. *Letter 506* (To his brother Theo), c.9 July 1888, R.G. Harrison, ed., 2001. http://www.vggallery.com/letters/619_V-T_506.pdf/ Last Accessed: November 18, 2008.

Van Voorst, Robert E. *The Koran,* In the *Anthology of World Scriptures*. Belmont, CA: Wadsworth Pub., 2006.

Wittgenstein, Ludwig. *Tractatus logico-philosophicus*. London: Routledge & Paul, 1961.

Zelanski, Paul, and Mary Pat Fisher. *The Art of Seeing*. Pearson: Upper Saddle River, 2007.

Index

Z

ABOUT THE AUTHOR

JASON K. SWEDENE is Associate Professor of Philosophy and Humanities at Lake Superior State University (LSSU) in Michigan. He has authored articles in Ethics and Emotion Theory, and a book, *A Philosophy of Moral Dilemmas: Why We Should Not Feel Guilty About Things We Have Done* (Lewiston: Edwin Mellen Press, 2007). Since 2005, he has served as Director of the LSSU Honors Program.

His Bachelor's degree in Philosophy and Psychology is from Le Moyne College in New York. He earned his Master's degree and doctorate in Philosophy from The University of Buffalo, New York. He lives with his family in the historic town of Sault Ste. Marie, Michigan.